The Pregnancy Handbook
for
Inexperienced mothers

Dennis E. Adonis

I0413354

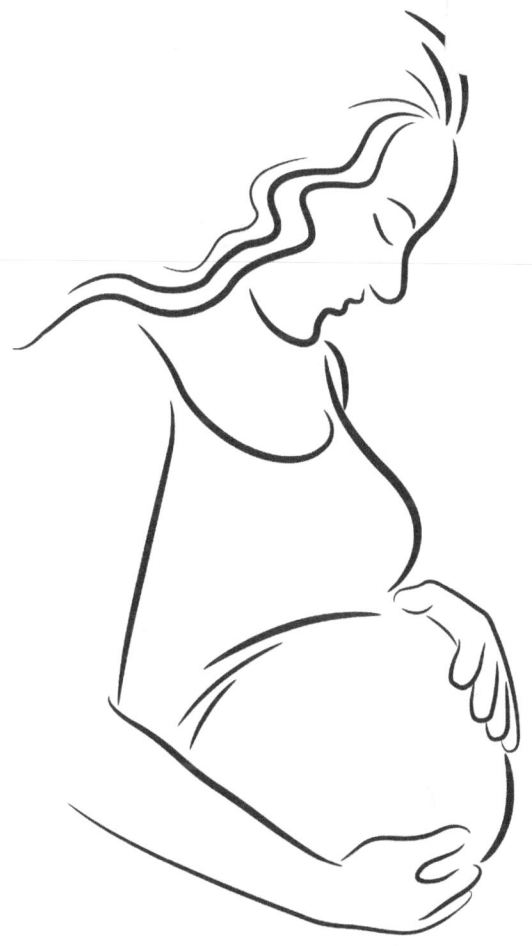

Mind Readers Publishing, Australia

Printed in the USA

Advisory

The Surgeon General advises that this book was written based upon the observed experiences, investigations, social analysis, maternal surveys, queries and opinions of the author. Therefore, it is to be used for discretionary informational purposes only.

And while the author have received material guidance from qualified medical doctors and other professionals within the medical fraternity, the information contained herein is not intended to be used in place of, or in conjunction with professional medical advice regarding pregnancy.

Furthermore, the author of this book is not a medical practitioner *(at the time of publishing)*, and does not hold himself out as one.

This book was written based upon professional medical guidance provided to the author by members of the medical fraternity. However, the Author and Publishers of this book may not be liable for any medical issues that may be claimed to have been caused as a result of the use of this book.

Prior to adhering to any literature-based medical advice, beginning any regimen or taking any medication, a pregnant mother must consult a licensed medical doctor for professional guidance, or to determine the best course of action for her individual situation.

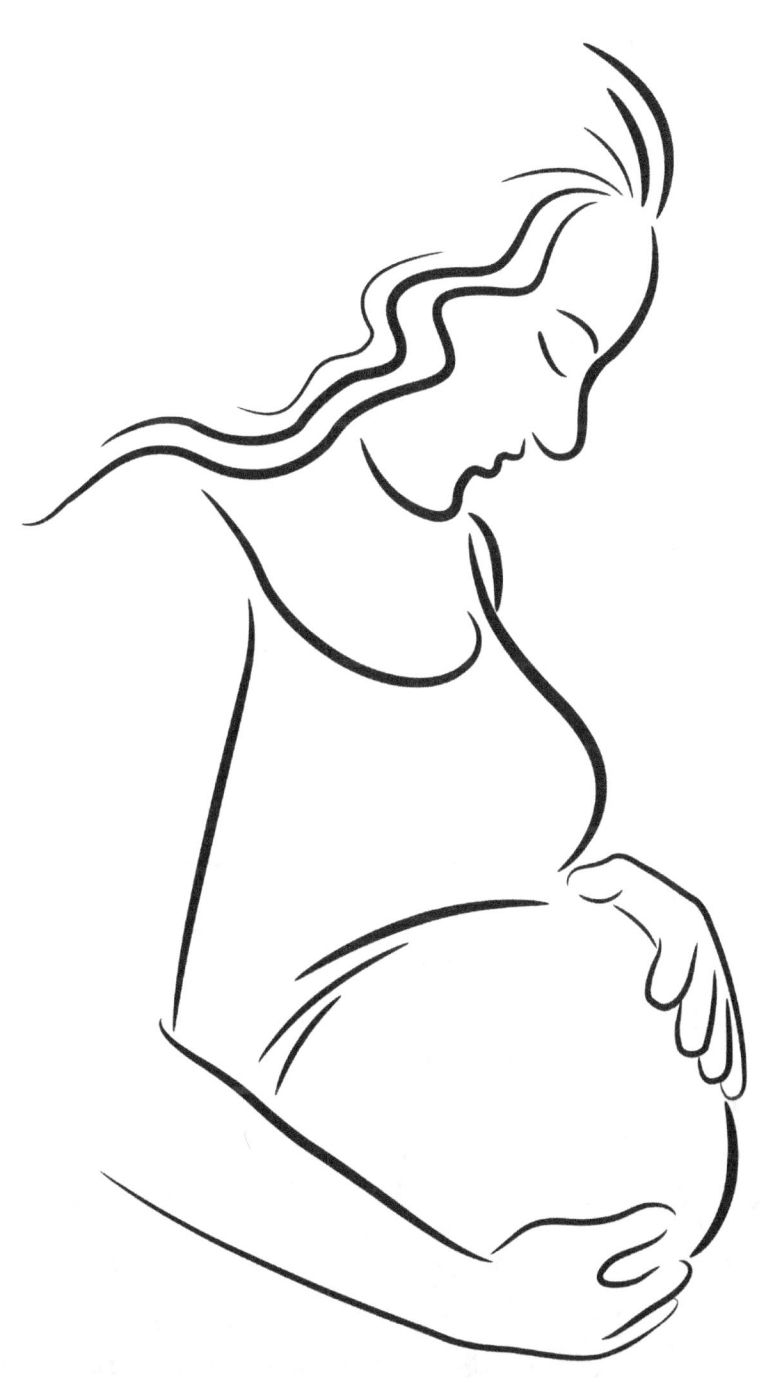

The Pregnancy Handbook for Inexperience Mothers:

Written & Compiled by Dennis E. Adonis

The Author may be available for reviews: email@dennisadonis.com

Acknowledgements

The Author (Dennis E. Adonis), would like to thank the following persons and entities for both their direct and indirect contribution to his work on this book; - The American Pregnancy Association, the National Institute of Child Health and Human Development, Johns Hopkins School of Medicine, Mayo Clinic, Oregon Health & Science University, the University of Melbourne, babycentre.com, whattoexpect.com parents.com, webmd.com, Jane Maloney for the PLR materials, and Mind Readers Publishing; all of whom have assisted me in some way during my quest to complete this book.

But most of all, I would like to thank the Almighty, and the mothers of my five children for the experience of fatherhood, as it has given me all of the inspiration to pen this book.

Published by: *Mind Readers Publishing – Melbourne, Australia.*

A first word from the Author

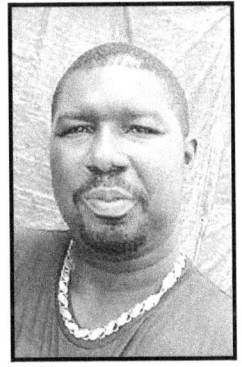

Pregnancy is arguably the most multi-complex element of human developmental biology.

It is the only means by which the human race *(and any other mammal)* can naturally secure mankind's continued survival and generational existence, for time infinite.

Realistically, if pregnancy should cease to exist at this moment, then just around a century from today, planet earth would have no human traversing its surfaces, and God's creation of the human race *(with a new Adam and Eve)* would have had to start all over again.

And even if you were to adore the theories of evolution and decides to look at the thought from that perspective, then it would take a few million years for anything close to today's human to ever evolve.

In either circumstances, such an occurrence would have been psychologically tormenting as science would have struggled (and arguably fail) to defy such a cursed derailment of nature.

But since such a biological event is seemingly impossible, the role and importance of pregnancy is often taken for granted, simply because it is a natural phenomenon that we all expect to happen.

However, from all social angles, the role of the woman and her importance to this very complex natural phenomenon of life is often overlooked by most of their spouses, even as the woman struggles to understand the pregnancy process herself.

In other words, an especially first time pregnant woman is often tasked with developing her own understanding of the pregnancy process, and finding answers to every single issue that pops up before her during her nine months of gestation.

On the other hand, men often inadvertently find it dumb when a pregnant woman says she don't know what is happening to her or can't explain why she is feeling a particular way.

Practically, in a man's shallow mindset about procreation, we expects a pregnant mother to know every single bits and pieces about her pregnancy without ever considering that she is going through a learning process; - sometimes over and over, as each pregnancy would present a different challenge.

From a father's perspective, and having been a witness to five pregnancies and the birth of five children, I was fortunate to learn about pregnancies five-fold because I was always inclined to pay keen attention to all five of those experiences, which is now complimented by over 14 years of research literature on pregnancies.

And even though I was able to learn a lot, I find that I was unable to effectively get my partner to comparatively peruse any pregnancy literature whatsoever because most of the books were either too cumbersome, medically technical, or did not address her core concerns from a lay man point of view.

After all, the average pregnant woman would not want to be juggling between a series of tormenting morning sickness' from a growing baby and bunch of 500 pages literature filled with medical jargons.

As such, I always felt that it is imperative for a concise book to be written for pregnant mothers who simply need a brief understanding of the pregnancy process, in addition to aspects of pregnancy that would matter the most.

But not being a medical doctor or a trained medical personnel, my initial efforts to personally and professionally compile such a book was stalled for over two years, until I sought literary support from some of the most prominent medical institutions, gaeneocologist and pediatric doctors from around the world, for almost the entire of 2013.

With their information support, and the first time utilization of a smaller percentage of private label content within the pages of this book, I was able to compile this concise literature on pregnancy *(from a lay man's point of view)* for primarily first time mothers requiring some maternity self-guidance.

As such, I trust that this book would be of material benefit to every would-be-mother that reads it, and that its objective of helping mothers-to-be to have a better pregnancy experience is achieved.

Dennis E. Adonis
Author

Table of Contents

What is Pregnancy?

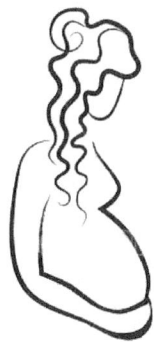

Pregnancy is the carrying of one or more embryos or fetuses by female mammals, including humans, inside their bodies.

In a pregnancy, there can be multiple gestations (for example, in the case of twins, or triplets).

Human pregnancy lasts for approximately 9 months between the time of the last menstrual cycle and childbirth *(38 weeks from fertilisation)*.

The medical term for a pregnant woman is genetalian, just as the medical term for the potential baby is embryo *(early weeks)* and then fetus *(until birth)*.

A woman who is pregnant for the first time is known as a *primigravida* or *gravida* 1: a woman who has never been pregnant is known as a gravida 0; similarly, the terms para 0, para 1 and so on are used for the number of times a woman has given birth.

In many societies medical and legal definitions for human pregnancy is somewhat arbitrarily divided into three trimester periods, as a means to simplify reference to the different stages of fetal development.

The first trimester period carries the highest risk of miscarriage *(natural death of embryo or fetus)*.

During the second trimester the development of the fetus can start to be monitored and diagnosed.

The third trimester marks the beginning of viability, which means the fetus might survive if an early birth occurs.

How Does Pregnancy Occurs?

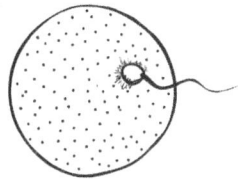

Before pregnancy begins, a female *oocyte* (egg) must join, by male *spermatozoon* in a process referred to in medicine as "*fertilisation*", or commonly (though perhaps inaccurately) as "conception."

In most cases, this occurs through the act of sexual intercourse, in which a man ejaculates inside a woman, thus releasing his sperm.

Though pregnancy begins at implantation, it is often convenient to date from the first day of a woman's last menstrual period. This is used to calculate the Estimated Date of Delivery (EDD).

Traditionally *(according to Naegele's rule, which is used to calculate the estimated date of delivery, or EDD)*, a human pregnancy is considered to last approximately 40 weeks *(280 days)* from the last menstrual period *(LMP)*, or 37 weeks *(259 days)* from the date of fertilization.
However, a pregnancy is considered to have reached term between 37 and 43 weeks from the beginning of the last menstruation.
Babies born before the 37 week mark are considered premature, while babies born after the 43 week mark are considered postmature.

According to Merck, the norm for human pregnancy is that it lasts 266 days from the date of fertilization. This is 38 weeks, or approximately 8 *Gregorian* months and 22.5 days, or 9.0 lunar months.

Counting from the beginning of the woman's last menstrual cycle, the norm is 40 weeks *(the basis for Naegele's rule)*.

According to the same reference, less than 10% of births occur on the due date, 50% of births are within a week of the due date, and almost 90% within two weeks. But it is not clear whether this refers to the due date calculated from an early sonograph or from the last menstruation.

Though these are the averages, the actual length of pregnancy depends on various factors. For example, the first pregnancy tends to last longer than subsequent pregnancies.

Nonetheless, an accurate date of fertilization is important, because it is used in calculating the results of various prenatal tests *(for example, in the triple test)*.
A decision may be made to induce labour if a baby is perceived to be overdue. Due dates are only a rough estimate, and the process of accurately dating a pregnancy is complicated by the fact that not all women have 28 day menstrual cycles, or ovulate on the 14th day following their last menstrual period.

Approximately 3.6% of all women deliver on the due date predicted by LMP, and 4.7% give birth on the day predicted by ultrasound.

The Odds Of Getting Pregnant And Age

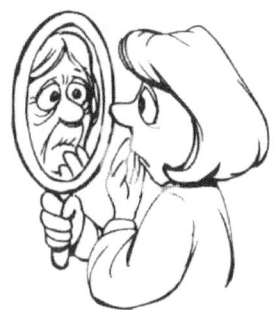

The odds of getting pregnant would certainly decline with age. The odds of getting pregnant are the greatest for a woman in her early twenties and then slowly decline with the passing years. Here are some numbers related to the chances of getting pregnant and age:

1. For ages early to mid-thirties - a woman in general will be about 15-20% less fertile.

2. For ages mid to late thirties - fertility will generally decline by up to 50%.

3. For women ages early to mid-forties - fertility declines by over 90%.

You may probably be wondering why do the odds of getting pregnant generally decline as the woman gets older.

Studies have indicated the reasons for fertility-decline are related to the quality of the woman's eggs as well as the quantity.

A woman in her lifetime will typically produce about 400 fully developed eggs (usually one per month) that are capable of becoming implanted in the uterus and causing pregnancy.

As these eggs get used up over thirty years or so and estrogen production slows so that the uterine and vaginal linings are no longer properly stimulated, pregnancy becomes less and less likely.

On the other hand, studies have found that the probability of causing pregnancy by a man in his late thirties declines by about 40% from the probability during his 20's to mid-30's.

However, a woman can increase the odds of getting pregnant by considering the following tips:

• Know your fertile time - ovulation generally happens about 14 days before your next period begins. For women with cycles of 28 days, that could make day #14 your most fertile for getting pregnant *(day #1 being the first day that your last period began)*.

• Monitor your basal body temperature - the slight elevations in your body temperature upon awakening each day will signal your most fertile time.

• Monitor your cervical mucus - ovulation will cause a change in the appearance and consistency of cervical mucus. Check yourself each day and you'll be able to see the 'egg-white-like' vaginal discharge that indicates your most fertile time.

• Adopt a healthy lifestyle - the odds of getting pregnant increases with the more healthy you are. Healthy living includes a sensible diet, nutritional supplements, adequate sleep, managing stress, exercise and weight management.

Planning to start a family, getting pregnant and pregnancy can be exciting, frustrating, fulfilling and without any certain outcome. Improving your health will add to the likelihood that you can become pregnant and have a healthy baby.

How to Get Pregnant

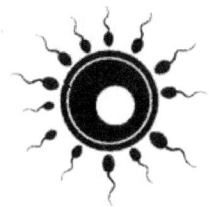

It seems that almost everyone has some advice to offer the couple who are having a little trouble getting pregnant.
Of course many women simply conceive more easily than others, and there's no doubt that some of that "good advice" can be helpful.

But simply relax is probably one of the more common pieces of advice and it's probably good advice. Studies have shown that stress can hamper efforts to get pregnant and some couples find that pregnancy occurs naturally once they stop worrying so much about what they are doing wrong.

But all that good advice should eventually give way to a trip to the doctor, if the couple are serious about having a child.

Many couples find that there are some simple answers to their problems and that solving those problems will allow them to get pregnant quickly.

Some people have found that a minor infection or illness was the culprit. In many cases, the person hoping to conceive may not have even known they were ill. A virus can send signals to the female body that pregnancy is not a good idea. A round of antibiotics or some other simple cure to a seemingly unrelated illness may be all it takes to get pregnant.

There are also many treatments and procedures that are relatively inexpensive, easy and non-invasive that allow couples to conceive, even if getting pregnant naturally isn't an option.

After all, not all fertility issues are serious, time-consuming and expensive. But if you're serious about becoming pregnant, one trip to the doctor may be all it takes.

By all means, take a little time to let nature run its course. But if you've been trying to become pregnant and it just hasn't happened for over a three year period, then it may be time to seek out some medical help.

When Is The Best Time To Get Pregnant (?)

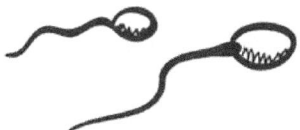

Every woman has a reproductive cycle that can make it easier for them to become pregnant if sexual intercourse is effected at the correct timing and correct days within that cycle.

The best days to get pregnant will generally be the time when ovulation occurs. To ensure that you act perfectly within the ovulation cycle, a woman should adhere to the following guidelines *(some of which had already been mentioned in a few pages earlier)*:

1. Know your most fertile time - generally, ovulation occurs about 14 days before your next menstrual period begins. That means if your menstrual cycle is a 28-day one, that could make day #14 your most fertile day (day #1 is the first day that your last period began). If yours is a 30-day cycle, day #16 could be the time to go for it. A 32-day cycle would have day #18 as one of the best days to get pregnant.

2. Track your basal body temperature - an inexpensive basal thermometer can be purchased and used to chart the slight elevations in your body temperature upon awakening each day that signal when is the best time to get pregnant. The increases in basal temperature may only be a tenth of a degree or so, but a basal thermometer can detect this kind of minor temperature change.

3. Monitor your cervical mucus - ovulation causes a change in the appearance and consistency of cervical mucus. By checking yourself each day, you'll be able to see the 'egg-

white-like' vaginal discharge that indicates ovulation and which are the best days to get pregnant.

4. Use an ovulation predictor kit - these inexpensive kits predict ovulation in advance so you definitely know when is the best time to get pregnant. This test has proven very accurate in detecting the increase in luteinizing hormone which usually occurs in women 24-48 hours before ovulation.

Are You Looking for Signs of Infertility?

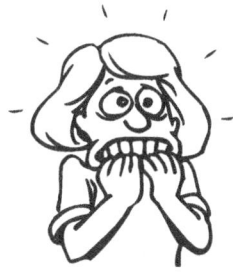

Trying to conceive is a difficult process for some people. The reason is that there are many factors involved in conception.

You cannot tell if you or your partner is infertile unless you visit a doctor.

There are a number of medical tests that your doctor can perform to detect infertility. There are also methods and products that the doctor can prescribe to help in conceiving a child.

One procedure a doctor can perform is to test the cervical mucus, because it plays an essential role in conception, as it enables the sperm to make it all the way to the egg.

The sperm are unable to do this if there is little or no cervical mucus present. Another factor involving cervical mucus is that it could be too acidic. It is necessary for the mucus to be alkaline. If it is acidic, it will kill the sperm before they reach the egg.

When a doctor checks the cervical mucus, he/she will look at the whether it is clear or curdled. If it is curdled, there is little to no chance of conception. If the mucus is clear and somewhat sticky, chances of conception are good.
Before you start to think about the possibility that you or

your partner might be infertile, make sure that you have been having unprotected *(natural method)* sex over a number of months, or up to two years.

Sometimes, conception can take a long time, even for couples who have no troubles with infertility.

Often, a couple may have unprotected sex for 8 or 10 months at about twenty times per month before conception takes place.
In other cases, it can take between one month to three years before pregnancy occurs.

Once you have given yourselves this waiting period, and conception still has not occurred, visit your doctor for what steps you should take next.

Try not to worry - focus on the many tests and procedures available to help you and your partner become parents of a beautiful baby.

Pregnancy Symptoms

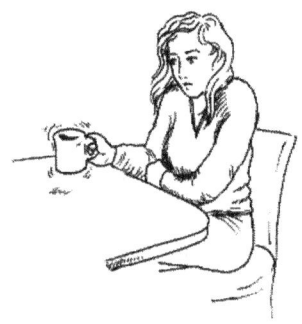

Missing the period is the most common sign and indication of pregnancy. However a variety of other reasons such as stress, illness, and weight fluctuations etc can also provoke late or missed periods.

Missing periods normally can also be a symptom of *polycystic ovary syndrome*, a condition in which periods can occur months apart. Hence one has to observe and examine the other symptoms to confirm pregnancy.

Another important symptom of pregnancy is the change in the size and feel of a woman's breast immediately after the conception.
Breasts would usually begin to enlarge to get ready for breast feeding and women claim that the breasts become sensitive and they experience a very sharp and twinkling sensation.

Another most common symptom of pregnancy is nausea and vomiting normally seen among women.
This is also known as morning sickness; - a feeling of sickness that is also experienced by most women from the fifth and sixth week of the pregnancy.

The morning sickness can start as early as two weeks from conception, while the degree of nausea, vomiting, tiredness and fatigue associated with morning sickness will differ from person to person.

Mostly these symptoms may disappear after a period of 3 to 4 months.

Frequent urination is also a common feature among pregnant women within 2-3 weeks after conception due to the reduction in the size of the bladder .

Drastic change in taste and smell is also another factor, compounded by craving for certain foods and suddenly hating certain types of food.

While all the above are pregnancy-associated symptoms only a clinical test can accurately confirm pregnancy, especially in its early stages.

One can confirm pregnancy by conducting the small home pregnancy test which determines whether a woman is pregnant by detecting the level of HCG in the urine.

You should note however that if the home-test result is positive you may need to make an appointment with a family doctor to confirm whether or not you may be pregnant.

Similarly a blood test at your local laboratory can also determine whether you are pregnant.

For more physical methods, an obstetrician can confirm the pregnancy by a physical examination, after a period of 4 to 6 weeks from conception.

The thickening of the vaginal tissues and the softening of uterus usually confirms pregnancy, via this method.

How Can Pregnancy Be Detected?

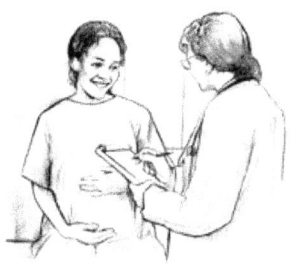

The beginning of pregnancy may be detected in a number of ways, including via various pregnancy tests which detect hormones generated by the newly-formed placenta.

A pregnancy tests basically detect the presence of *human chorionic gonadotropin*.

Clinical blood and urine tests can detect pregnancy soon after implantation, which is as early as 6-8 days after fertilization.

Home pregnancy tests are personal urine tests, which normally cannot detect a pregnancy until at least 12-15 days after fertilization. Both clinical and home tests can only detect the state of pregnancy, but cannot detect its age.

In the post-implantation phase, the *blastocyst* secretes a hormone named *human chorionic gonadotropin* which in turn, stimulates the *corpus luteum* in the woman's ovary to continue producing *progesterone*.
This acts to maintain the lining of the uterus so that the embryo will continue to be nourished.

The glands in the lining of the uterus will swell in response to the *blastocyst*, and capillaries will be stimulated to grow in that region. This allows the *blastocyst* to receive vital nutrients from the woman.

When To Take A Pregnancy Test

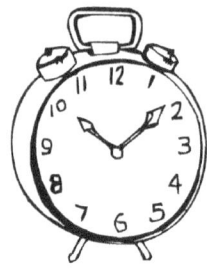

A pregnancy test, as the name implies, is simply a test used to determine whether or not a woman is pregnant.

When to take a pregnancy test is important, because if you test too early in your pregnancy, there may not yet be enough of the pregnancy hormone in the urine to provide a positive test result, even though you are already pregnant (by a few days).

And if you test too late, you might not be able to make proper provisions to determine the way forward or even to effectively evaluate the circumstances as it relates to your health and readiness for a baby.

If you're wanting to know when to take a pregnancy test, the timing may depends on the type of test to prefer to take, among other minor independent factors.

Basically, there are two types of pregnancy tests. These are the urine test and the blood test.

Both tests looks for the hormone that is only present if a woman is pregnant. This hormone is called 'human chorionic gonadotropin', also referred to as 'HCG'.
Blood tests can detect HCG as early as 6 to 8 days after you have ovulated.

On the other hand, urine tests can detect HCG about 14 days after ovulation.

Generally, you can test a basic home-test if you feel that you have been exposed to sperm insemination or if you are having symptoms at least two weeks from your last date of inseminated sex.

Many women would first try using a pregnancy test (at home) that will test the urine to determine if they are pregnant. Home pregnancy tests are convenient, inexpensive and are private.

These can be found at most major retail and/or drug stores and can provide quick results.

Because these are amateur tests (meaning they are not performed by a licensed medical doctor), there is always the possibility of a false reading.
But if the directions are followed correctly, however, the accuracy rate is quite respectable.

Before seeing a doctor, many women want to have an idea as to whether or not they are pregnant, which is why an at home pregnancy test (urine test) is a very popular first choice.

The urine test should be done using your first urine when you awake in the morning.

Most of the home pregnancy (urine) tests will be 90% accurate if you wait and do the test yourself one day after your missed period is due, or about two weeks after your time of unprotected sex.

If you have a positive home pregnancy test result, you should then see your health care provider at the earliest opportunity.

Your health care provider will then confirm your home test result with a more reliable blood test plus a pelvic exam.

However, if you feel that you are pregnant but the home pregnancy test is negative, repeat the test again in a week if you still have not had your period, or is having pregnancy concerns.

And if you are still getting negative test results but sincerely thinks that you may be pregnant, please see your health care provider right away.

During the visit, a physician will relay the determination of pregnancy or the absence thereof and, if necessary, will provide additional information for expectant moms.

It can be difficult to realize the symptoms of pregnancy for first-time moms-to-be, which is why it is important to learn about the possible signs of an early pregnancy as discussed earlier.

But as a reminder, these early pregnancy signs may entail an increased sensitivity to certain foods and/or smells, recurring morning sickness, fatigue, exhaustion and mood swings.

It is important to have a pregnancy test following the onset of any or all of these symptoms because a positive result may mean that a new change in lifestyle may be in order.

When the results are negative
- Invitro Fertilization - The Male Point Of View

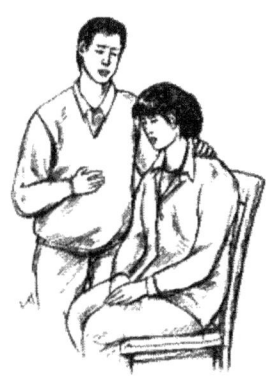

For some people who are not desirous of becoming pregnant, a negative result from a pregnancy test may be a joy to them.

However, a negative result (especially a repeated one) can be a devastating factor for other couples who may have been desperately trying to have a baby to compliment their union.

But for some of couples, sexually related medical conditions or an unrealized vaginal bacteria may very well be the culprit that is preventing natural fertilization.

In other scenarios, it may be a scenario that is mostly attributed to the male partner.

In those cases, the affected couple may opt to conceive via *Invitro Fertilization*.

In-vitro fertilisation (IVF) is an assisted reproductive technology by which an egg *(taken from the woman's ovaries)* is fertilised by sperm (in a lab) outside of the body of the woman, and then surgically reinserted back into her uterus so that it may evolve into a fetus, and in essence, a child.

IVF may be the most effective form of assisted reproductive technology in use today.

The procedure can be done using your own eggs and your partner's sperm. However, this option is usually retained by couples when all other treatments or methods to get a woman pregnant had failed.

It is often considered a last resort because it can be time-consuming, expensive and invasive.

For those couples who decide to pursue *Invitro fertilization*, the time leading up to the fertilization will be very process orientated - as there will be consultations, evaluations, forms, literature and a lot of listening. At times it may seem overwhelming and frightening.

As the male participant in the process, the man's involvement will be largely in a support role, as most of the work that will need to be done will be with the female partner.

To help make the process as easy for his partner, there are a number of facts that a man has to keep in mind and a number of actions he can take to help keep his female partner's spirits up and to help her in the necessary steps to achieve a successful fertilization.

- You and your partner may struggle with the fact that you are unable to conceive by natural means. However, keep in mind - although it may not be a natural form of conception, the end result and the end goal of the process is the same - a healthy child.

The two of you are merely trying to maximize the possibility of a healthy & successful pregnancy. Talk through this point and be open to each other's feelings.

- There will be a lot to absorb about the process, so take notes and do your research to get a better understanding of IVF.

- Some of the medications required for the process will need to be administered via injection. A male partner can offer to administer the shots if his partner is not comfortable doing so, and keep in mind that she will most likely be very sore in the injection spots because of repeated shots.
A little tender loving care will help keep both parties confident and comfortable.
Also, a heating pad may help during periods where the woman's abdomen is very tender.

- You will be asked to take very specific medications, at very specific times and will need to consult with the doctor on a somewhat frequent basis, often times on very short notice.

Therefore the male partner should make sure that he keeps his schedule as free as possible so you can be assist with transportation and medicine administration as needed.

- The female partner may experience emotional mood swing because of some of the meds. One minute she might be sitting at the table reading the newspaper, the next she is crying about something unrelated. The male partner must be prepared, be supportive and remember that her mood will return to normal in time.

Invitro is not an easy process, especially compared to natural fertilization. But with care, cooperation and a willingness to unite, the entire experience can be a very rewarding one.

Outside of *Invitro*, several other unconventional methods can be employed to integrate natural born children into the family, such as surrogation, etc.

When the results are positive

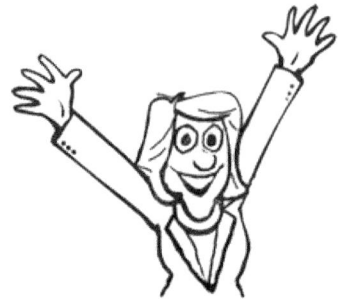

Getting pregnant and pregnancy itself can be a wonderful event that is equally complex, satisfying and exciting for couples who wants to have a child or children.

So if on your first or on your humpteen try, your pregnancy tests shows a positive result, then it will be time for you to start preparation for an often unpredictable and sometimes challenging journey that usually amass the stage of conception right through to delivery.

A positive pregnancy result can also bring both joy and anxiety, but would certainly bring about a change to your life, health, and social order depending on a multitude of factors that usually follows after a woman would have discovered that she is pregnant.

But of course if the result is positive from a home test, then the first thing you may need to do is promptly consult with your health care provider for a professional test, and joining of a maternal care regime.

Announcing Your Pregnancy

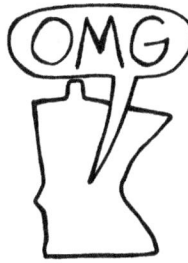

When a woman finds out that she is pregnant it becomes difficult to think about anything else. This can result in the woman being anxious to announce the exciting news to other people specially their partner.

There has always been a lot of controversy on the best time to make an announcement about the pregnancy. But the variation seems to differ mostly because of cultural and other reasons.

When choosing how and when to make an announcement about your pregnancy it is necessary to know the advantages and disadvantages of proper timing. Moreover one can choose creative ways to reveal the secret.

For a woman who may not have had a well crafted education, a career, the financial strength, a family-approved partner, her own accommodation, evidence of solid independence, or is dependent upon their parents or relatives; - announcing her pregnancy can sometimes be a nightmare or a family disaster that can often transcend into a division among those approving and those disapproving of such a step.

Nonetheless, you may want to at least try as quickly as possible to put certain mechanisms in place that can help you to deal with criticisms and objections to your choice of becoming pregnant.

Therefore, the first and most important thing to do is to ensure that your partner fully supports your pregnancy, and is putting systems in place to ensure that no financial or other hiccups will beseech you.
After all, being pregnant and not having a willing man by your side to face your friends and family can be the worst repeating dose of nightmares to come.

But outside of his support, the most important above all is your own strength and desire to proceed with the pregnancy.

Once you feels that you are strong and ready enough, then you can choose different methods to gradually get the news across to your families and friends, depending on their perceived demeanor upon hearing such an announcement.

Generally, it is mostly the decision of the mother as to when and whom she wants the big news to be announced.

In any case, you should be careful about whom you tells.

Telling your partner first would be best thing to do since it will immediately bring a sense of belonging and a bond with the child, in addition to making you feel supported.

After the spouse, the other people who should know are the parents *(if they are not going to eat your eat off, and depending on your relationship with them)*. They can help in future planning, offer advice and rejoice like no other person.

But surprisingly most couples usually prefer to break the news first to their best friends, then to someone else who they hope may somehow get it to the hearing of their parents.

Naturally, not all women or couple have the strength to stand up in front of their parent and say mom *(or dad)* I am pregnant.

Sometimes the thought of the hurricane that would follow after you said that and the long list of questions and criticisms that will follow, might be too much to take.

But whatever you do, you may want to be mindful of how and when to share the news.

If you are someone with a good sense of humour and really do not care what people thinks, then here are some fun ways to make the announcement to friends and family

#1 - Show up to a family gathering wearing a dress or shirt that announces your state. These days there are a ton of shirts out there with clever sayings like; - "Baby on Board," "A Bun in the Oven," or something related to the pregnancy. The moment you walk in or take off your jacket everyone will figure it out without you ever having to say a word. Now, get ready for the tears and excitement. You'll be answering a ton of questions too.

#2 If you already have children you may want to call the grandparents up and tell them that the next Christmas they may want to add one more name to Santa's list.

If this is the first grandchild, you may want to get a bracelet link for your mom that reads, "#1 Grandma" or grandparent t-shirts. This will not only be a great present for them but something they will cherish and love forever.

No matter when you spread the news it can be a lot of fun, just think creative and let the pieces fall. You may even want to try catching all of it on video, so think ahead and be prepared for the many reactions at various forums.

However, in some instances, sharing the news early or late have their own advantages and disadvantages.

If one shares the news early, the main advantage is that there may be; -

- A lot of support from near and dear ones.
- A lot of time is available for advice and to choose the best medical professional.
- overwhelming support in case of a miscarriage.

The main disadvantage of breaking the news early is that there may be; -

- criticisms and disagreements with some relatives including parents depending on your age and educational prospects.
- overwhelming advice to the stage of stressing you out.
- a lot of explanation needs to be done in case of a miscarriage.
- depression from a miscarriage when everyone was anticipating a perfect pregnancy.

But whether you choose to announce it or not, everyone would end up knowing at some point, unless you remains in a state of concealed hibernation.

Furthermore, you still need to start taking steps to care for yourself and the unborn baby, in addition to dealing with the many challenges that pregnancy brings.

How To Care For Your Body During Pregnancy

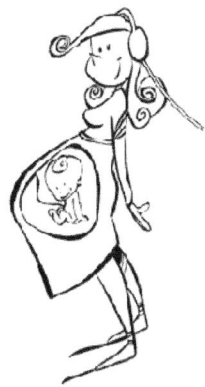

Being pregnant and following a healthy lifestyle is more important than ever. It is crucial to understand what steps you can take to keep you and your baby in good health.

Prenatal care is one of the vital factors that ensure a smooth pregnancy.
The first checkup should occur during the first 6 to 8 weeks of your pregnancy, when your menstrual period would have been approximately 2 to 4 weeks late.

Primarily, proper nutrition is one of the best ways to enjoy a happy pregnancy. Because you're eating for two, it's doubly important to consume healthy foods and stay away from things that may harm your baby as it develops.

When you're pregnant, dieting and cutting calories is not a good thing - you will need to take in about 300 more calories a day to ensure you and your baby are properly nourished, especially as your pregnancy progresses. Caloric intake, however, can vary from woman to woman.

For thin women, and women carrying twins, you may be required to consume more than 300 extra calories. Or, if you are currently overweight you might need less. No matter what, you'll need to contact your healthcare provider to determine what's best for you.

Of course, pure calorie consumption is not the only goal - you need to make sure that what you eat is nutritionally sound. Nutritious foods contain the essential vitamins and minerals that contribute to a baby's growth and development.

Although a healthy diet is fundamental to caring for your body during pregnancy, it's actually quite simple to integrate healthy living into your daily life.

Maintain a well-balanced diet by following basic dietary guidelines. Lean meats, fruit, vegetables, whole grain breads and low-fat dairy products are all essential to maintaining good health.

Real, healthy food will provide your body with much-needed nutrients. At the same time, during pregnancy certain essential nutrients are required in higher-than-normal amounts. For example, calcium, iron, and folic acid are especially essential in the diet of a pregnant woman.
Although your doctor may prescribe vitamin supplements, your diet still needs to contain nutritious food to provide your body with most of its nourishment.

On a normal basis, women need 1,000 mg of calcium per day, but during pregnancy, calcium consumption should rise in order to keep up with calcium loss in your bones.

You can get calcium from a wide range of food products, including low-fat dairy products such as milk, cheese, and yogurt; orange juice, soy milk, and cereals that are fortified with calcium; dark green veggies such as spinach, kale, and broccoli; as well as tofu, dried beans, and almonds.

A pregnant woman requires 27 to 30 mg of iron per day because iron is used by the body to make hemoglobin, which is what helps red blood cells carry oxygen throughout the body.

A lack of iron leads to a dearth of red blood cells, meaning the body's tissues and organs don't receive enough oxygen. With a baby on board, women need to pay extra attention to their iron intake.

Iron is found in both plant and animal matter, but the body absorbs it more easily from meat sources. The following are some foods that contain a good amount of iron: red meat, dark poultry, salmon, eggs, tofu, enriched grains, dried beans and peas, dried fruit, leafy green vegetables, blackstrap molasses, and iron-fortified breakfast cereals.

Many people have already heard about how important folate (folic acid) is for a pregnant woman.

For pregnant women, or those planning on becoming pregnant, it is recommended that you take 0.4 milligrams of folic acid every day.

Many women choose to supplement their diet with vitamins in addition to any folic acid intake they receive from food.

It has been found that consuming folic acid one month before and during the first 3 months of pregnancy reduces the risk of neural tube defects by 70%, which is why it is considered so critical.

The neural tube is formed during the first 28 days of pregnancy, which is usually before a woman even realizes she's pregnant, and it eventually develops into the baby's brain and spinal cord.

Lack of sufficient nutrition, particularly a lack of folic acid, may result in a neural tube defect such as *spina bifida*.

To remain healthy while pregnant, it's also key to drink plenty of fluids. During pregnancy your blood volume increases, so drinking plenty of water is the best way to avoid dehydration and constipation.

Exercise is a great way to feel great throughout an entire pregnancy. There's no reason to stop physical activity once you become pregnant; in fact, dietary guidelines suggest that you take 30 minutes or more each day to work out at a moderate pace.

During pregnancy, regular exercise prevents excessive weight gain, reduces problems such as back pain, swelling, and constipation, improves sleep, increases energy, promotes a positive attitude, prepares your body for labor and lessens recovery time after labor.

Proper sleep is another factor in maintaining health and comfort during pregnancy. Pregnancy can take its toll, and after a long day you will feel more tired than usual. As the baby grows bigger, it will be more difficult to sleep, but try to sleep as best you can - it will do wonders for how you feel!

Following a healthy diet, getting enough sleep, exercising, and drinking plenty of fluids are all important to your overall well-being during pregnancy.

If you strive to eat nutritious food and maintain a positive attitude during the course of your pregnancy, the good moments will definitely outshine the difficult ones.

Food Cravings During Pregnancy

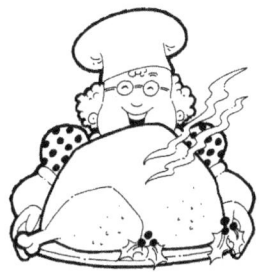

Do pickles and plain rice sounds good to you? How about red peppers and ice cream? If these do, then these are meals that would often be enticing to a pregnant woman who would not had ordinarily eat such a strange combination as a delicacy.

More than three quarters of all pregnant women experience cravings at some point. The most common cravings are for sweets, dairy products and salty foods although there are some weird cravings for chalk, raw meat, uncooked rice and many other strange foods.

As bizarre as some cravings can be, they are mainly perfectly safe.

There are old wives tales that insinuate that what you crave could be a good indication of the sex of your baby. According to those old beliefs; - if you are craving sweets you are having a girl; if you crave meats or cheeses, it is believed you are having a boy.

Cravings are something that most women love most about pregnancy. However, it is when a woman is craving dirt or clay that an alarm should go off.
If you should find yourself craving dirt, soil, or chalk call your doctor right away. Not only could these be harmful if you do

eat them, but chances are they are a sign of iron-deficiency anemia.

Most doctors believe that cravings can be nutritionally based. That is to say the cravings are a message from your body on what it needs to eat.

If you are craving salts foods it could be because your body needs more sodium as your blood volume increases. If you are craving fruit, your body might need more vitamins C. But the problem is that sometimes the message gets lost on the way to the woman's brain.

As such, you may find yourself craving something sweet. And instead of getting berries or fruit, you find yourself gulping down snicker bars by the cart full.

Cravings can be the downfall of your weight gain especially if the message is getting scrambled.

Fortunately, there are some steps that you can take to help curb your cravings.

- For starters, eat a good breakfast. Eating a good breakfast can prevent cravings later in the day.

- You also want to try and make wise choices by looking for healthier alternatives. If you are dying for potato chips try eating some soy crisps.

- Instead of ice cream, try frozen yogurt. If you feel like candy is calling your name, snack on some frozen grapes.

- If you want something salty, try pretzels, or even rice cakes to satisfy that urge.

- A good substitute for soda would be some fruit juice mixed with sparkling water.

- Another good practice is to consider eating small rather than big. That is to mean that if you are craving chocolate, you do no need to reach for a king size bar. The small snack size bar will satisfy your craving just the same. If you want fried chicken, have just one piece; just do not eat the whole bucket.

In actuality, there is nothing wrong with indulging in a few of your cravings as long as you know not to over do it.

Moreover, giving in to your cravings during pregnancy does not make you a bad person and it is not something you should beat yourself up about and feel guilty about.
Cravings are a normal part of pregnancy and denying yourself all the time might make you resent being pregnant.

Indulge when you want to, but just make sure you make wise choices and do everything in moderation.

Eating Well For Your Baby

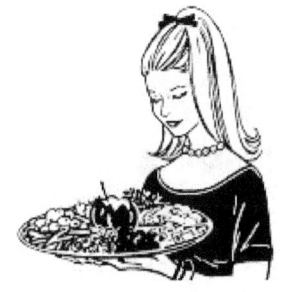

The next nine months are going to be an exciting time, not just for you but for your growing baby.

Think of all the things a baby has to accomplish in only nine short months.

They start as a single cell and then divide at an enormous rate. Their organs develop, the heart forms and starts beating and all five senses form.

Basically your baby goes from a little blob that can't be seen with the human eye into a seven, eight, nine or even ten pound adorable newborn baby.

In order for your baby to develop as healthy as possible, your diet should play a big part. This is because your baby is going to receive all the vitamins, minerals, protein and fluids that he or she needs to grow and develop from the diet you intake.

The best thing you and any other pregnant mother can do for your growing baby is to eat as healthy as you possibly can, because eating well will certainly benefit your baby.

First, eating right is going to help your baby's organ development. Your baby only has a short time to develop vital organs such as their heart, liver, lungs, and kidneys. Eating a diet that lacks vitamin D or calcium can interfere with your baby's bone and tooth growth.

Furthermore, eating too lightly throughout pregnancy might stop your baby from growing as it should in your uterus.
Too light-eating would cause you to measure behind for where you should be in your pregnancy, and would similarly cause your baby to be seriously underweight.
This may be bad for you because small babies are at a greater risk for health problems once they are born.

On the other hand, eating too much can cause your baby to grow too big too fast. Babies who are measuring ahead are at a greater risk for delivery complications. Babies who are too big usually can not be delivered vaginally without the assistance of instruments such as forceps or a vacuum.

Some research has been done that shows what you eat during pregnancy can affect your baby's eating habits down the line.
Babies can taste and get use to the flavors from food that makes its way into the amniotic fluid.

It is quiet possible that your baby will have a preference for certain foods before they even take that first spoonful of solids. Therefore, by making sure your diet contains a lot of vegetables and fruit can help ensure that your baby will enjoy eating that healthy category of food went the time comes.

Also, as hard as it may be to believe, some studies have shown that what you are eating can contribute to your baby's personality.

Research has shown that babies born to mothers who were under-nourished tend to smile less and are drowsier compared to those who are healthy.

Also, studies have shown that moms who consumed enough omega-3 acids during their final trimester have babies who showed healthier sleep patterns than other babies.

Lastly, your baby's brain needs you to eat healthy especially during the last trimester.

Unlike the rest of your baby's organs, the brain has its greatest growth spurt during the third trimester.

This is the best time to eat protein, calories and omega-3 fatty acids. These will ensure optimum brain development.

Eating Well For You During Your Pregnancy

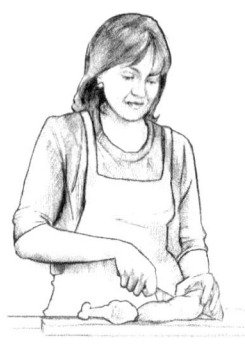

Eating healthy throughout your pregnancy is the greatest gift you could give your unborn baby, but there are also a lot of rewards in it for you too.

It is common for many moms to forget that they also benefit in eating healthy through out their pregnancy.

What you eat has a direct effect as to how well your body copes and recovers from all the physical changes it goes through.
It also helps with the physical and emotional challenge of carrying and delivering a baby.

The truth is, most pregnant women rarely walk around all nine months with that rosy glow everyone talks about.

During the first three months, some moms walks around a nasty shade of green and in a hazy fog thanks to the tiredness they feel for those first three months.

The second three months are a little better, and mothers are no longer green but can deal with other issues such as varicose veins and leg cramps.

The third trimester, they are back to the hazy fog again and have other issues such as swelling and heartburn just to name a few.

Some of these experiences can be avoided with a good diet.

Eating foods that have some complex carbs can help reduce your tiredness and staying away from fatty foods will help with the heartburn.

Research has shown that pregnant women who eat healthy throughout their pregnancy usually have a safe and uncomplicated pregnancy.

Studies have also shown that some pregnancy complications such as *preeclampsia* or high blood pressure can be directly related to deficiencies in a pregnant woman's diet.

High amounts of sugar and polyunsaturated fats increase this risk as well as having a low intake of vitamin C, E and magnesium.

Perhaps for some women one of the biggest benefits of eating healthy during their pregnancy is that it could help them during labor and delivery.

A well balanced pregnancy diet has been said to help prevent preterm labor, which is labor before 37 weeks. A good diet can also help you cope with labor and delivery better.

Any woman who has given birth knows how much energy it takes to endure hours of contractions and sometimes hours of pushing.

Eating healthy will ensure that you have the energy and the stamina to get through your little one's delivery.

Eating Well to Deal With Morning Sickness

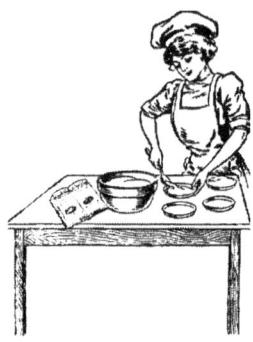

There are a few women out there in the world who sail through their pregnancy without so much of glimpse of queasiness. But the rest of them have no such luck.

Chances are you are the type of woman that the mere smell of what use to be your favorite food now sends you running to throw up at the nearest toilet sink.

Even the mere sight of steak can send you heaving and just thinking about eating that salad turns you greener than the romaine lettuce it contains.

You will probably fumed at whoever named it "morning sickness" when all pregnant women know it is more like an all day sickness.

Interestingly though, there are different degrees of morning sickness. Each woman and each pregnancy is different.

A woman can spend the first three months of her first pregnancy over a toilet and unable to look at any sort of vegetable or meat. However, the situation can be different with her second pregnancy which can entail only a few spurts to the bathroom and hardly any aversions.

The good news is that morning sickness is usually only a temporary experience for pregnant mothers.

Most women would start feeling better between their 12th and 14th week of pregnancy. But as hard as it is to eat healthy during this period there are some things you can still do to help ease your discomfort.

1 - For starters, eat often. It has been shown that an empty stomach tends to make your morning sickness even worse. This is why so many pregnant women feels so bad when they first wake up.

Having to burn lots of energies overnight to supplement their babies, the waking mom would have had nothing in their system; which means their stomach's acids are going crazy since nothing is there to soak them up.

The trick to this is to eat often. Try eating around six mini meals a day and make sure you have plenty of snacks. Make sure you eat often in bed too.

Before you go to bed for the night have a snack that is high in protein and in carbs such as nuts and raisins, yogurt and bread stick or a cheese and crackers.

Keep a stash of crackers or ginger cookies by your bed and make sure you have one before you even think about getting out of bed in the morning.

You will always want to eat mainly carbs and protein, but you can also stick with crackers or fruit to give you some comfort during those first few months.

Other good snacks are pretzels, saltines and whole grain toast. For fruits stick with melons and bananas.

For your protein add a little cheese or some nuts to your snacks or any time you are feeling a little green.

Yogurt is also an excellent choice when fighting morning sickness.

2 - Make sure you drink your water. If you are vomiting it is essential that you stay hydrated.

Making sure you stay hydrated is probably more important that making sure you eat those first few months.

Becoming dehydrated can cause lots of problems for you and your little one. So make sure you drink at least 8 glasses of water or juice throughout the day.
You can also suck on ice chips or fruit juice popsicles if you are having problems keeping liquids down.

The most important thing to keep in mind those first three months is not to beat yourself up if you cannot eat as healthy as you would like to. You will still have plenty of time to make up for it after you get through this storm.

Just make smart choices when it comes to what you eat and snack on and that will pave the way for when you can eat as a normal person.

Eating to Prevent Heartburn

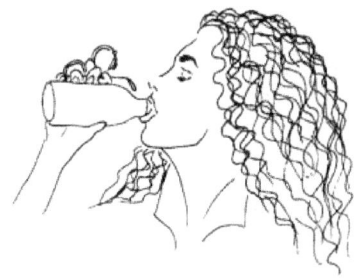

Heartburn does not just affect those who are high stressed or love their spicy foods.

Pregnant women suffer from heartburn too. You will find that as your pregnancy progresses, antacids tend to become your best friend.

Actually, heartburn has nothing to do with your heart. It is a condition that occurs when the acid from your stomach leaks up into the esophagus.

Heartburn is very common during pregnancy. In fact one in four women experience heartburn during their pregnancy, particularly during the third trimester.

The reason is that your baby has grown a tremendous amount and your uterus has moved up and is now putting pressure on your stomach.

This would then crowd the digestive tract and allows acids to travel back up the esophagus.

There is an old wives tale that if you have bad heartburn, your baby will have a lot of hair. Of course there is no proof in this but it is a fun thing to believe in.

On the reality side, there are things that you can do to help prevent heartburn during pregnancy.

You can start by taking your time while you eat. Not only will you enjoy your food better but your stomach will not have to work as hard to digest your food.

You also want to try eating early and eat at least two hours before you go to bed at nights so that your body has plenty of time to digest your food.

Keep your meals small. Stick with eating six small meals throughout the day. Large meals tend to stuff up your stomach which is already extra squashed thanks to your uterus.

A stuffed stomach makes it more likely that some of the food along with stomach acid will make its way back up the esophagus.

Also, make sure you keep your fluids and solids separate. Too much fluid mixed with too much food can distend the stomach which can aggravate heartburn. You may also want to eat sitting up, and not while lying down. And if you are having a bed time snack make sure you are propped up by pillows.

Your weight also plays a part in how much heartburn you may experience. The heavier you are, the more pressure you are placing on your esophageal sphincter. This is another reason why your pregnancy weight gain should not be too much more than the recommended amount.

Another good step is to figure out what foods cause your heartburn. Once you figure out what foods causes your heartburn, you can cut them out of your diet.

Some foods you might want to steer clear of are highly seasoned spicy foods, soda, tomatoes sauce, chocolate, and some citrus.

Greasy foods are also a big contributor to heartburn. Cutting out greasy fried food is certainly going to help with your heartburn prevention.

When all else fails, take some baby-safe medications for your heartburn. Tums and Rolaids are said to be perfectly safe to take during pregnancy.

If you are not comfortable taking any over the counter medicines, then you can try some natural ways such as eating a handful of almonds.

Almonds are a stomach settler and might help with your heartburn. Another natural remedy is a tablespoon of honey mixed with milk, which is a favorite for preventing heartburn.

Like with some pregnancy discomforts, heartburn is one that can be avoided as long as you take the right steps and eat properly.

After all, even without suffering from a lot of heartburn, your baby can still be born with a full head of hair.

Eating to Beat Pregnancy Fatigue

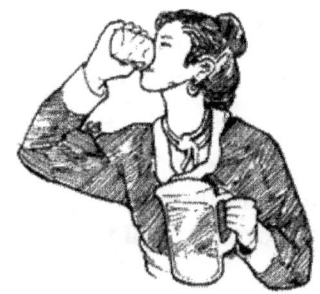

Ask any pregnant woman who is in her first or third trimester how they are feeling and the answer will almost always be "tired".

One of the first clues that many women have that they may be expecting a visit from the stork is the fact that they find themselves droopy eyed in the middle of the day for no reason.

You may find that doing a simply task such as walking around the block leaves you desperate for an afternoon nap.
The energy you use to have is now faced with the challenge of growing a baby and your body is hard at work. You are also producing more blood, using more water and nutrients and have a higher heart rate and metabolism because you are pregnant.

While the best defense method against the tiredness you will face is to get more sleep, there are also some healthy food choices that you can make to help you get through your day if you do not have the opportunities to take naps.

First, adjust the size of your meals. Anyone who eats a large meal is going to feel tired afterwards regardless of if they are pregnant or not.
Therefore, taking a big meal while being pregnant is going to be much worse, since most of your energy is going to be used towards digesting the meal; thus you will of course feel sluggish and drained.

Therefore, you should eat smaller meals and eat more often.

Do not skip lunch. There are many people who skip lunch thinking they will make up for it by having a big dinner. This is bad when you are not pregnant but it's even worse when you are pregnant.

You need that midday meal to help refuel your body. As with your breakfast, you should keep it filled with whole grains and protein.

Have a whole grain pita and stuff it with chicken salad and add a side of grapes or an apple.

Plan to eat most of your calories during the day. A pregnant woman needs an extra 300 calories a day throughout their second and third trimester.

However, during the the first trimester such a large volume of calories will not be needed .

You should eat these extra calories throughout the day in the form of healthy snacks such as nuts, cheese, veggies and dip.

Do not save your biggest meal until the end of the day. Your body needs these calories to help you get through your day.

Steer clear of the quick sugar fixes like candy and soda. In the end these will only make you more tired.

Lastly, make sure you are getting enough iron. Eat iron fortified food such as spinach and lean red meat to keep your energy up.

There are times when extreme fatigue could be the symptom of an iron deficiency and you might need an iron supplement also.

Besides eating well, make sure you get plenty of rest even if this means pushing your bedtime up and giving up those late night TV talk shows.

As any parent of newborns will tell you; - get your rest while you still can *(before your baby venture into the world)*.

Foods to Avoid While You Are Pregnant

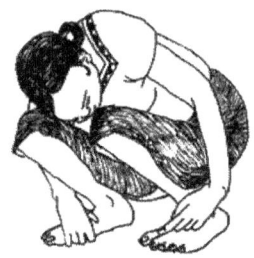

Almost every woman knows that during pregnancy they should cut back on caffeine; they should not smoke, drink alcohol or spend time in any hot tubs.

However more and more studies are being done to see if pregnant women should avoid certain foods for the duration of their pregnancy.

It is essential that pregnant women eat a well balanced meal at all times to provide their growing baby with the vitamins, nutrients and minerals that the baby needs to grow.

However, there are some foods though that pregnant mothers may need to avoid due to the risk they pose to not just to the mother, but also to the growing baby.

For starters, raw meat and undercooked meat needs to be avoided due to the risk of *toxoplasmosis* and *salmonella*. This means no more rare steaks, or rare burgers, or animal-based sushis.

Pregnant women should take caution and make sure that all of the meat that they eat is well cooked.

Cold deli meat should also be avoided because of the risk of *listeria*. This bacteria can cross the placenta and can cause an infection or blood poisoning to the baby. However, deli meat can be reheated until it is steaming and this will help reduce the risk.

Listeria bacteria can also be found in other foods such as some categories of soft cheeses including brie, feta, and gorgonzola. These cheeses are commonly manufactured with unpasterized milk which is often known to contain listeria.
Therefore, pregnant women need to make sure that any soft cheeses they are going to eat are made with pasteurized milk.

Fish has always been a subject of debate for pregnant women. While some forms of fish contain essential nutrients that are needed by the baby, others contain a high level of mercury.

Any fish with a high level of mercury such as shark, swordfish, king mackerel, tilefish and fish used in sushi should be avoided throughout pregnancy.

Studies have linked mercury to developmental delays and in some cases brain damage to babies.

Fresh Tuna also contains a lot of mercury, but canned, chunk light tuna has a lower amount of mercury and can be eaten in moderation.

Raw shellfish should also be avoided throughout pregnancy.

Raw eggs or anything containing raw eggs is a no no during pregnancy, since there is an obvious potential for exposure to *salmonella*.
This means no raw cookie dough, no brownie mix, and certain homemade sauces such as hollandaise, Caesar dressing and blue cheese dressing.
When dining in a restaurant, it would also be wise not to for ask any sauces or dressings that contain raw eggs.

Exercise During Pregnancy

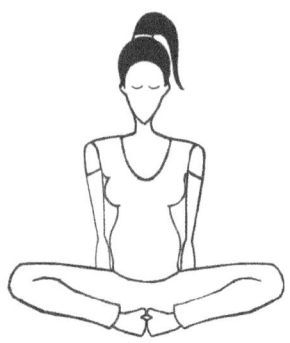

For some women the thought of exercise during pregnancy is as appealing as a tooth extraction without novacane.

In their minds they have a nine month excuse to keep avoiding their gym routine.

The first three months they are battling morning sickness and exhaustion. The next three months they are beginning to show. The last three months are so uncomfortable that walking ten feet to the bathroom is pure torture. So there is no way they will want to walk on a treadmill for ten minutes.

On the other side of the coin, there are some women who do not let pregnancy stand in their way of exercise. These are the women we might actually see teaching a class at the gym, or speed walking through the neighborhood with their protruding bellies.

Most pregnant women however fall somewhere in the middle and that is just how their doctors like it.

Exercise comes highly recommended when pregnant. Not only does it help control weight gain, but some women swear it helps with delivery also.

But while exercise is good for pregnancy, there are some things to keep in mind in order to protect yourself and your growing little one.

For starters you need to keep an eye on your heart rate as you are working out. Letting your heart rate rise to high could be dangerous to your little one especially in your first trimester.

You want to maintain a steady heart rate and should do the talk-test throughout your workout to make sure you are at a safe level. The talk-test is when you talk during your workout.

If you are having a hard time talking and wind up huffy and puffing more than getting out actual words, then you are working too hard and need to take it down.

Most doctors recommend that you work at a pace where talking is challenging but still doable.

Pregnancy is not the time to try out new exercise routines. This means that you should not try the new spinning class that your gym offers. Stick with the routine you have already been doing and that your body is use to.

You may also find that you have to make some modifications to some of your exercises as your pregnancy progresses.
If you are a runner, a modified low impact jog throughout your first trimester is fine but once you enter your second trimester and begin to show, your jog has to be brought down to a walk.

For those of you who love sit ups, crunches and floor push-ups, you can continue to do these up until you hit about 14 weeks or so. After that time period, no floor exercises are recommended.

If you do not have any sort of exercise routine in place before you get pregnant, this still does not give you a free pass.

Almost every doctor will tell you that walking is a great exercise for any pregnant woman who are not high risk.

Walking at least thirty minutes, three times a week is a safe way for a pregnant woman to stay active.

Walking is something you can do throughout all three trimesters, though you might find yourself moving at a slower pace by your third trimester.

Another great plus to walking, especially as you approach your due date, is that walking can actually bring on labor. Many doctors will advise their patients to walk, walk and walk some more in the weeks leading up to their due dates to get things rolling.

Some women who have walked throughout their entire pregnancy have an easier delivery and recovery period.

So while strenuous exercise is a not a recommended item, pregnancy is no longer a good excuse to stop moving.

Gaining Weight Too Fast During Pregnancy

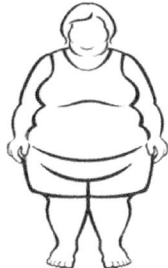

Any obgyn will tell you that the recommended weight gain for pregnancy is 25-30 pounds. Some women will gain more, some will gain less.

Too much weight gain can surely increase your chances of a C section and put you at risk for being overweight after.

But how can you tell if you are gaining too fast during your pregnancy?

Some doctors say that if you put on more than 3 1/2 pounds in your first trimester and are of a normal weight, you are putting weight on too fast.

If you are overweight and put on more than 2 pounds, you are gaining too fast. Keep in mind though that even if you gain a lot in your first trimester, it doesn't necessarily mean you will gain a lot throughout your whole pregnancy.

Some women gain a lot in the first trimester because morning sickness has them only able to eat carbs and nothing else and still end their pregnancy gaining no more than 25 pounds.

If however you find that your weight gain is still not slowing down once you enter your second trimester, there are some tips you can try to help slow it down.

First, cut out the useless calories. It is never a good idea to diet while you are pregnant. But if you are gaining too much you do need to slow down the rate at which you are gaining.

Apply some basic calorie cutting strategies such as using skim milk instead of whole milk, taking skin off your chicken and grilling or broil instead of frying or sautéing.

You will also want to cut out most of your sweets. These are empty calories that are providing no nutritional value to you or your baby.

Next, cut down on the fat you are taking in. Look at what you are eating and if it may have hidden fat in it.
Some salad dressings can be loaded with fat, so you might want to try putting your dressing on the side.
Watch how much oil you use when you are cooking or when you are going out to eat and stick to good oils such as extra virgin olive oil.

Get active! You could be gaining weight faster because you are not active.

As long as your doctor gives you the go ahead, start a walking program. Walking is one of the best things you can do for your body and your baby.
Not only does it help with your weight gain, but some women and doctors swear that walking throughout most of your pregnancy could help ease the pains of childbirth.

If you cannot walk due to weather conditions you might want to look into joining a prenatal exercise class.

Lastly, pay attention to what you are eating. Many pregnant mothers don't pay attention to what they eat and may be overeating without even realizing it.

How many times have you sat on the couch watching a movie and decided to have some potato chips only to realize that you have eaten the whole bag? Try to keep all your meals at the table and take your time while eating.

Even though you are eating for two, gaining just enough weight will not only make delivery and recovery easier for you, it will also make getting the weight off after pregnancy an easier task.

Gaining Weight Too Slowly During Pregnancy

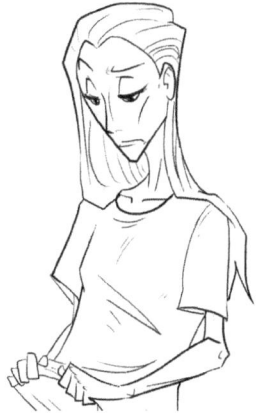

Just as gaining too much weight can be harmful to you and your baby; not gaining enough weight can be harmful also.

There are quite a few pregnant mothers out there who are so terrified at gaining weight that they eat next to nothing during their pregnancy.

And if you are one of them, then please do not do this, since you could be depriving your baby of the vitamins and minerals it needs, while increasing the chances of having a small and nutrient deficient baby.

Babies who are underweight at delivery are at a greater risk for health problems than babies who are of average weight at delivery.

If you find that you have gained nothing during your first trimester, do not worry, since your baby's needs are relatively tiny at that point.

Some women do not gain anything during those first three months and some even lose some weight thanks to morning sickness.
However, it is when you are in your second and third trimesters that you should make sure you are gaining weight accordingly.

If you find that you are not gaining as much weight as you should, you should try to fatten up your diet.

Increase your fat intake by a serving or two. This will increase your calorie intake but won't decrease your appetite. Nonetheless, do not increase your fat by more than a serving or two.

If you are one of the few lucky women who do not gain weight easily, you might not want to eat foods with the lowest amount of calories. You can still eat healthy but you may want to up your calorie intake.
Try eating avocados and more cheeses along with some beans too. Indulge in some snacks also.

Make sure you have a decent amount of calories but not so many calories that may ruin your appetite for your next meal.

If you are not allergic to peanuts, try some apple slices with peanut butter or some whole wheat crackers which some low fat cheese slices.

Take some time out of your busy life to relax, because not gaining enough weight could be a sign that you are doing too much. By being too busy and too active, you could be burning up the calories you eat instead of using them to nourish your baby.

You also want to make sure you eat after a workout to replace the calories you just lost. If you are working while you are pregnant and it is a stressful job, make sure you take the time out of your busy day for lunch and snacks.

Throughout all of this, check in with your doctor. Your doctor may want to run some tests to make sure that you do not have a thyroid condition or any other undiagnosed medical problem that might be keeping you from gaining weight.

You may also want to keep track of what you eat so you can show your doctor and talk about any changes that might need to be made to your diet.

How to Cope With Food Aversions

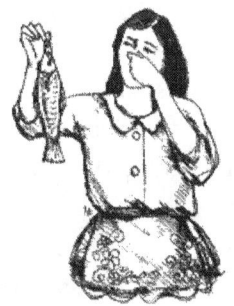

Do you find yourself suddenly feeling queasy at the thought of the left over pasta or pizza that you could not get enough of the other night?

If so, you might be going through a pregnancy phase called "food aversion".

Food aversion is when you or or body suddenly starts rejecting the smell, scent, and taste of food and drinks that you would have normally consumed.

Food aversions are a normal part of pregnancy and the flip side to food cravings.

Nearly eighty five percent of all pregnant women suffer from food aversions.
This experience appear in the first trimester and usually trigger that part of pregnancy we call morning sickness.

Some women find that they disappear by the start of their second trimester right around the same time morning sickness disappears. Other women find that their food aversions stay with them throughout their entire pregnancy, while other women would find that foods that they had developed aversions to throughout the pregnancy continues to be averse to them even after they deliver.

Just like with food cravings, your hormones are more than likely to blame for your food aversions.

Some experts believe that just as food cravings are your body's way of telling you that you need a certain food, food aversions are your body's way of protecting you from eating anything that can harm your baby.

This might be why a lot of women report that they experience aversions to alcohol and coffee.
The theory is still under debate though because so many pregnant women are turned off by food that is also healthy for them and their babies.

Nonetheless, try not to put up an all out fight against potentially healthy aversion. Consider it a blessing if the mere thought of your normal morning cup of coffee turns your stomach upside down.

In such a case, cutting back on caffeine will be a walk in the park for you.

Overall, if you find that you have aversions to healthy foods, try to work around it as best as possible.

On the other hand, do not force yourself to eat foods that you have aversions to. Instead, you can try to look for alternatives.

For example, if you find that the thought of salad or anything green is revolting to your sight or stomach, try and drink some vegetable juice, as an alternative.

While drinking vegetable juice is not the same as eating vegetables it may have its benefits if you can't look at your veggies.

You should also try eating different color veggies like peppers or carrots.

If it is proteins like fish and chicken that makes you sick, you can get your protein in other forms, such as yogurt, or eggs.

Alternatively, you can ask your partner to try and hide the meat in your dishes. For example, they can mince cooked chicken and then stir it into a casserole, or mix some fine-chipped seafood into a pasta dish.

This way you can still get your protein in, minus the risk of getting sick.

Just like with morning sickness, do not beat yourself up if you cannot eat as healthy as you would like while you are dealing with food aversions.

Chances are once you enter your second trimester, the aversions will disappear and you can resume eating a wider variety of foods.

Overcoming First Trimester Symptoms

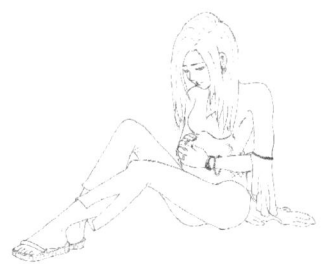

In general, pregnancy is divided into three trimesters. And each one has its own nature.

But for starters the first trimester of your pregnancy can be the most tormenting, and one of the most crucial time when you should be most careful with your fetus.

While we have discussed quite a few symptoms and associated scenarios earlier in this book, now might still be a good time to quickly recap them in a more concise manner before we move on to some other aspects of this subject matter.

So here we go again (with a list of first trimester symptoms);

1. Morning sickness - Nausea and vomiting are two common symptoms of early pregnancy. Hot drinks, crackers, and fresh fruits are great choices for relieving both.

2. Frequent urination - The growing of uterus would cause some pressure on your bladder., which would cause you to be going to the restroom more often.

3. Tender breasts - The increasing hormone lets your breasts become more sensitive, fuller and heavier than usual. This time you may replace your bra with a more comfortable one.

4. Uncommon Exhaustion - Don't push yourself by working too hard. Try to get some rests whenever you feel fatigue.

5. Increased craving - Acquire nutritious and balanced food intake. Make sure you and your baby are well nourished.

6. Bad moods - The change of hormones in your body causes your moods to switch as well. Mild exercises can help your moods. Moreover, just think that it's a preliminary change and challenge you'll have before and after your baby arrives.

Some of you may not recognize that you're pregnant until it reaches five to six weeks from your last period. But soon when you find it out, it's best to think which health care provider you'll go to for a routine check-up.

Enjoying Your 2nd Trimester!

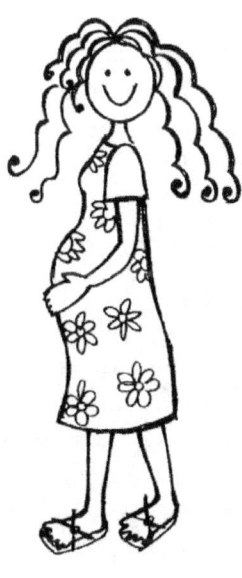

Congratulations! Your pregnancy now comes to the second trimester, which is within weeks 13 through 27. Your morning sickness has faded away gradually by now. This means, you should be feeling better than before.

The second trimester is actually the stage when you experience the most enjoyable moment with your pregnancy.

You'll feel energetic and full of vitality. You can do a lot more than when you were in the first three months.

However, this does not mean you can do anything you want. You still need to be cautious about what you do and avoid doing too many activities.

To help you to pull through your second trimester of your pregnancy, you can take note of the following tips and guidelines;

1. Control your appetite. Compared to the previous trimester, it's improving now. Try not to overeat and compromise your diet, since this can lead to you becoming overweight. Get balanced nutritious food instead of fast food.

2. Handle leg cramps by straightening and lifting up your legs for several minutes. If you get cramp, move your toes upward and hold for a few seconds.

3. Carry out 'low impact' exercise. Getting pregnant does not mean you do not need exercises. They are even needed at this time. Swimming, yoga, and walking are good exercises for pregnant women. Ask your hubby or friends to join you.

4. Perform Kegels to strengthen pelvic floor muscles. Simply squeeze the muscles for a few seconds and let them relax just like when you stop and start urine flow. Do it several times a day as trained muscles can make labor easier.

5. Enjoy love-making with your husband. These months are the most comfortable time for both of you to do it.

Another incredible element of your second trimester is the fact that you will start feeling little snaps of movements by your growing baby in your womb.

Vaginal bleeding during pregnancy

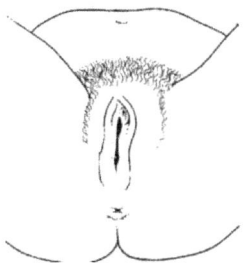

Before, we dig into the topic of vaginal bleeding during pregnancy, we may want to first establish that there is a difference between bleeding and vaginal spotting.

In actuality, spotting is when you notice a few drops of blood every now and then on your underwear. It may not even be enough to cover a panty liner.

Spotting is a normal occurrence during the earlier phases of pregnancy, but can also be a sign of an ectopic pregnancy *(a pregnancy where the fertilized egg develops outside the uterus),* which can be life threatening for a woman if left untreated.

On the other hand; bleeding is a heavier flow of blood.

With bleeding, you will need a liner or pad to keep the blood from soaking your clothes.

Vaginal bleeding during pregnancy is referred to any instance(s) where there is discharge of blood (or spotting) from the vagina.

This can occur at any time between the period of conception (when the egg is fertilized) to the end of your pregnancy.

However, its occurrence is more common during the first 20 weeks of pregnancy, and may only be experienced by about 3 out of every ten pregnant women.

Vaginal bleeding often leaves a number of clueless mothers-to-be in a state of disenchantment, since they are uncertain about what may be causing it or whether it is an indication of a potential miscarriage.

Various professional indications have established the most common causes of vaginal bleeding, which may be because of;

- Having sex
- An infection
- The fertilized egg implanting in the uterus
- Hormone changes
- Other factors that will not harm the woman or baby

However, you may have a medical emergency if the following factors are associated with your vaginal bleeding experience;

- Heavy bleeding
- Bleeding with pain or cramping
- Dizziness and bleeding
- Pain in your belly or pelvis

After all, the above more seriously associated elements may very well be a sign of; -

- A miscarriage, which is the loss of the pregnancy before the embryo or fetus can live on its own outside of the uterus. Almost all women who miscarry will have bleeding before a miscarriage.

- An ectopic pregnancy, which may cause bleeding and cramping.

- A molar pregnancy, in which the pregnancy does not form properly.

However, if it just a simple case of minor vaginal bleeding, then there are a few steps that you can take to avoid unnecessary bleeding, all together.

How to prevent bleeding during pregnancy(?)

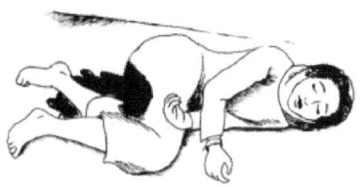

Taken from the experiences of several women who would have encountered vaginal bleeding during pregnancy, you may want to consider the suggestions listed below;

1. Be careful with constipation. The strenuous push of the bowel muscles can easily cause the bleeding. Eat more vegetables, fruits and drink more water to prevent constipation.

2. No heavy lifting. Don't lift staff heavier than 5 pounds. Seek others' help when you need to move something.

3. Bend at the knees to pick up something. Don't lift abruptly. Bend at the knees slowly and stand up slowly too.

4. Lie down/get up slowly. Don't jump onto/out of the bed. A good way is before going to bed, go to the edge of the bed, lie down slowly with your side and then turn onto your back. Similarly, when you want to get out of the bed, turn to your side and get up slowly.

5. Don't wear high-heeled shoes. Wear soft and flat bottom shoes.

6. Always hold on to something when you climb stairs, especially downwards.

7. Be careful with doing exercise. Avoid those fast-paced exercises.

8. The last but not the least is, being relaxed and happy. After all, stress can provoke hormone imbalances and lead to vaginal bleeding.

Maternity Clothes: *Dressing For Your Pregnancy*

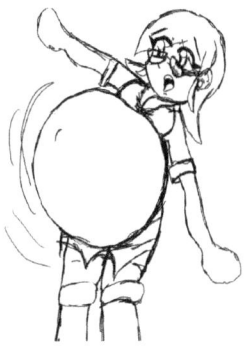

The first time anyone would actually see any real physical proof that you are pregnant is during your second trimester.

This is the time when a small baby bump is actually beginning to show, as your little one begins to accelerate their growth rate within your womb.

And as nature would have it, your tummy may need to expand itself gradually outward to make room for your growing baby.

But while nature may be busy doing its job to expand your tummy, you would discover that most of your clothing that you were accustom to wear during pregnancy is not feeling comfortable on you anymore.

Furthermore, some of your regular clothing might even make you look awkward and poorly attire since those clothes would not had been designed for you in that state.

Therefore, during your second trimester it would have been time for you to start switching your main wardrobe to a maternity closet.

A wide variety of special maternity clothes are usually available at major retail stores and other virtual maternity boutiques online.

You don't have to forcibly fit yourself into ordinary clothes and feel uncomfortable all the time. You can pick from a range of maternity clothes according to your preferences and occasion, as listed below;

● *Intimate apparels*

Now, pretty lingerie is most women's desired wear. It has to be comfortable as well as pretty.

During pregnancy comfortable lingerie is a must for you. You don't have to wear your regular size and feel stuffed and stilted at all. A wide range of comfortable, yet attractive underwear is available for expecting mothers these days.

Cotton nursing bras are the most comfortable bras for you during this period. They are stretchable and are also available with multiple hook options so that you can wear them according to your requirements. These bras can also be used after the pregnancy period, as they are stretchable and are available with hooks for making the right adjustments for breast-feeding.

Maternity thongs are also available quite readily in the market. These sit comfortably below your belly. They are made super stretchy and soft. They allow your panties to grow for the nine months, giving you an appropriate fit. Maternity thongs are available as 3 pack seamless thongs and 4 pack seamless thongs as well.

Bikini panties are also amongst the must-have maternity apparels to buy for a mom-to-be. These are made up of cotton and are available in fresh colors. These maternity panties are available in floral, striped or solid prints of panties. These can provide you with essential comforts for your underwear.

● *Maternity T shirts*

Wearing T-shirts gives a sense of comfort and relaxation for every mum-to-be. You can also buy and wear T-shirts during your pregnancy.

Now you don't have to sit and gaze at one of your lovely T-shirts just because it doesn't fit you anymore. You can buy dozens of lovely maternity T-shirts for yourself.

You can buy a ¾ sleeve ruched T-shirt, which allows you to look smart and leave you feeling cool. Long sleeve T-shirts with branded bottom and scoop neck would fit you just fine.

V neck tees, short sleeve crews, short sleeve tees, polo tees and sleeveless v-neck Ts are available in maternity sizes for you to choose from, So wear them out and about and feel good about your new life role and looks.

● *Jeans*

Would you get jitters, if you were asked to wear jeans, during the maternity period?

Does it sound too absurd to wear jeans with a huge belly?

And you also think that it is too uncomfortable to be worn during the pregnancy period?

Not any more. Jeans as maternity clothes are made for your comfort.

You can wear these specially designed jeans and feel confident as well as comfortable. These maternity jeans include an all around stretch panel and come in all cuts and sizes. They are available as panel free waist jeans with boot cut leg.

Tab waist stretch crosshatch jeans are also comfortable options for you.

● *Skirts*

Skirts are women's most sought after apparel. Maternity skirts are available readily in the shops and you can pick the one of your choice from the internet as well.

So wear maternity skirts without any hesitation. You can pick the one from the readily available options such as long denim skirts, denim button fly skirt, dark denim knee skirt or contour waist short stretch denim skirt.

How to buy maternity clothes

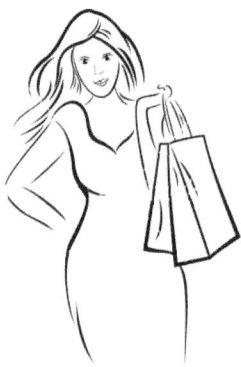

So now you know that you can wear all types of clothes during your mom-to-be phase. But hold on. You need to consider some aspects before you start shopping for maternity clothes

You should buy maternity clothes which give you extra room. The primary comforts should focus on belly and bust.

You should even consider plus size maternity clothes if you are expecting twins.

You should also buy your basic items made up of stretchable fabrics.

It is advisable that you only buy one or two bras at a time. This is for a reason that your size will increase and change periodically during the course of nine months.

You should buy nursing bras during the final months of your pregnancy. The fitting of these bras should be perfect.

If you find it too uncomfortable to be out shopping during this stage, you must check out the maternity wear available on the Internet.
The net is the best place for you to get the right kind of maternity apparel for all occasions without having to leave the comfort of your home.

Preserving Health And Beauty In Pregnancy

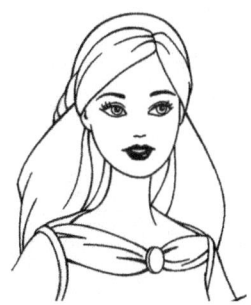

Most women think that it's okay to stop exerting effort into looking beautiful during pregnancy; - but it's not.
Pregnancy is a time when your hormones are in a rage. It is easy to be overwhelmed by new feelings, sensations, and changes in your body that make you feel not in control. But taking care of your pregnant self lets you be in control and preserve your health and beauty.

It's not easy to look in a mirror with disheveled hair and dry, blotchy skin. It's also frustrating to try and fit yourself in your pre-pregnant outfits.

Get rid of the idea that this is normal. What's normal is a pregnant woman embracing and enjoying her pregnancy by taking care of her body, her health and beauty.

Studies have shown that babies born of happy mothers are healthier -- they are heavier, more active, and agreeable.
They also absorb more nutrients from their first feedings which are essential for their nourishment.
Happy mothers are also found to produce better-quality milk for their babies.

Negative emotions increases the risk of developing post-pregnancy depression. This affects how a mother bonds and cares for her newborn.
As such, the best way to ward off this negativity is to preserve your health and beauty.

First, follow a healthy diet under the specifications of your doctor. Do not assume that the diet your other pregnant friend follows is right for you.
Your health and beauty needs are unique, since you may have deficiencies or skin care needs, which your friend's diet cannot address.

Secondly, take supplements and vitamins according to your doctor's instructions. Never take drugs or any form of medicine without your doctor's approval. It may have adverse effects on your baby.

Thirdly, exercise lightly to avoid gaining excess weight. Expectant mothers normally gain 15-20 pounds; anything higher than that can give you a difficult delivery.

Fourth, get adequate sleep and rest. Nothing is more stressful than sleepless nights because of hormones and restlessness. Make up for lost sleep during the day; your body will tell you when it needs some shut-eye.

Of course, a pregnant woman's health and beauty are not limited to her physical needs. Her emotional and psychological well-being are just as important.

You know that nothing boosts your confidence than being thought of and complimented as beautiful.
You can easily get that goddess feeling again through modern maternity fashion.

Contemporary maternity designers are coming out with new designs that showcase your pregnant body rather than hiding it. Take advantage of your fuller cleavage and wear lower necklines.
Show off your pregnant belly in stretch tops that hug your curves in solid colors. Avoid hiding in busy prints and opt for simple, understated accents and accessories.

Change your hairstyle -- pregnancy is a perfect excuse to try the new pixie cut. Keep your posture straight and your feet pretty in fun flats and funky mules.

Health and beauty are essentials for a pregnant woman. Take care of yours and you will be better-equipped in caring for your baby.

Treat your pregnancy as your time to shine with natural health and beauty.

Staying healthy and beautiful during pregnancy is not only easy; it is the best thing you can do for yourself and your baby.

Stretch Lines and Pregnancy
- Causes and Prevention

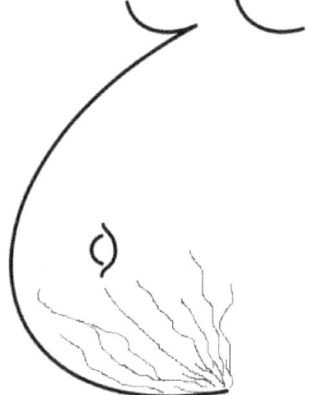

Stretch marks; *Striae Gravidarum*; The marks of pregnancy; - Call them what you will. But they are the one thing that all women dread, as it will begin to show itself gradually from the latter stage of your second trimester.

But what are stretch marks anyway? And why do they occur?

Well, the reason lies in the anatomy of the skin. The skin has two layers – a thin upper layer called the *epidermis*, and a thicker, lower layer called the *dermis*.

Scattered in the dermis are fine protein filaments called *elastin,* that, like a piece of rubber band, are capable of stretching on being pulled.

But just as a rubber band can stretch only so far and no further, these elastin fibres can also be stretched only to a certain extent. Because if stretched further, they will snap.

As may be obvious, the increasing bulk of the uterus during pregnancy causes the skin to stretch to a great extent and thus causing the elastin fibres to become torn.
The torn elastin then produces scars on the skin called *Stria Gravidarum* or stretch marks.

● *These marks occur on the lower abdomen of all pregnant women, right?*

Well, right and wrong. Because while they appear on most pregnant women, it does not necessarily appears on all of them.

Furthermore, it is not always restricted to the lower abdomen. Practically, stretch marks may generally occur when the skin is stretched within a very short period of time, even in other situations outside of pregnancy. Nonetheless, it may occur:

- In the lower abdomen in pregnancy.
- Along the sides of the breasts in pregnancy or in obesity.
- On the upper thighs during rapid weight loss or weight gain.
- Occasionally even on the inner sides of the upper arms to people who are not pregnant or obese.

● *But can stretch marks be prevented?*

Thankfully, the answer is yes, to a certain extent.

Although some women are genetically prone to develop stretch marks, it has been noted that athletes and women accustomed to heavy, physical labour get very few or no stretch marks. This is regardless of whether their female relatives have stretch marks or not.

The reason for this is that that these women have very well-developed and strong abdominal muscles.

These muscles can easily take the weight of the growing uterus and prevent it from pressing forward on the skin – rather like wearing a strong muscular belt under the skin. The skin is thus stretched less; - less elastin fibres are damaged, and there are fewer stretch marks.

Again a supple, healthy, well moisturized skin is capable of stretching more without any lasting damage. So if a woman can strengthen her abdominal muscles and keep her skin healthy and supple, there is less chance of her developing stretch marks.

● *But How Can You Develop muscles and Keep Your skin Moisturized?*

There there is probably just one natural thing that you can do to beat stretchmarks, and help to make your protruding tummy look healthy and beautiful.

And that one thing is gentle exercises.

Gentle exercises for the abdominal muscles can be started as soon as pregnancy has been confirmed or even as pregnancy is being planned, so that the tummy muscles can be nurtured into preparation for stretching.

These gentle exercises are few in numbers, but can certainly do the trick.

Exercise 1: Standing erect, raise both arms above the head. Bend forward slowly to touch your toes. Hold the position for a count of 100. Then slowly straighten up. Do this exercise at least once daily.

Exercise 2: Standing erect, raise both arms above the head and clasp your hands. Now bend slowly to your left as far down as you feel comfortable. Hold for a count of 10. Straighten up slowly and then bend to your right. Hold to a count of 10. Straighten up. Exhale as you are bending and inhale while straightening up. This makes one set. Do at least 3 sets once daily.

Exercise 3: Stand straight with feet about 12 inches apart. Place hands on your back at the waist. Slowly bend back, as far back as you feel comfortable. Hold to a count of 10.

Straighten up. Now bend forward slowly, hold the position to a count of 10. Then straighten up. Exhale as you are bending and inhale while straightening up. This makes one set.

Do at least 3 sets once daily.

These three exercises will strengthen the abdominal and back muscles as well as gently stretch the skin. They can also help to improve your posture during pregnancy.

But while gentle exercises is good, you may also need to consider a good diet, complimented by the application of direct skin care efforts to your tummy in order to yield better results.

❏ *Caring for the skin:* Keep the skin moisturized by applying oil – olive oil, coconut oil, almond oil or any good baby oil – thoroughly over the skin of the abdomen, hips and thighs. Massage it in with sweeping upward strokes.

You can do this before you exercise so that the oil is properly absorbed as the skin is stretched during exercise.

This will make the skin supple and healthy and capable of stretching without damaging the elastin fibres.

❏ *A Good Diet:* Take a good diet with lots of fresh fruits and vegetables and adequate liquids. And do not forget your daily vitamins.
This will ensure a healthy and supple skin.

● *But what happens if the stretch marks have already occurred; How do I get rid of them?*

The good thing about stretch marks is that they fade over time.

When they are first formed, they are reddish or purplish, but later they become thin silvery or gray and may not be visible at first glance (particularly on darker skin individuals).

The elastin and collagen growth can be stimulated to some extent by cocoa butter, Vitamin E, wheat germ oil and lanolin.

But to remove the marks completely, laser surgery, blue light therapy and other surgical treatments are the only options.
Many creams and lotions available on the market also claim to be able to remove stretch marks but have yet to be medically proven and accepted.

Pregnancy And Massage Therapy

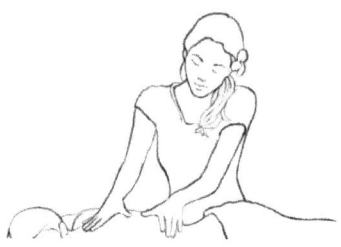

When you are pregnant, your body is under tremendous pressure. Everything hurts, everything aches.
But how can you get relief from this tension and stress.

Massage after all is out of the question, isn't it? Well maybe not.
Because of its importance and benefits to mothers, there are many massage therapists today who are specialize in Prenatal Massages.

In essence, a prenatal massage is a less rigorous and maternal specific physical therapy that promotes relaxation, soothes the nerves, and relieves strained back and leg muscles in expectant mothers.

Because of the fact that it targets pregnant women, most of the techniques that a prenatal massage therapist uses will concentrate on a woman's, neck, back and pelvic regions. These are of course the areas most often negatively affected by a pregnancy.

Comparing to regular massage procedures, one of the big difference in a prenatal massage will be your position.
Since you cannot and should not lay on your stomach, you will most often be laid on your side with pillows for support.

While there are special tables designed to allow room for a pregnant tummy, most therapists will prefer to have you rest on your side.

If you are modest, don't worry, your therapist will be able to customize the massage to your specifications while respecting your personal limits.

The benefits of massage during pregnancy are numerous. When you are under stress, your body produces stress hormones. Stress hormones that you produce will be felt by not only you, but also your baby.

By reducing your stress, through massage, you can increase the safety of your baby. It can also ease your muscular aches and pains that can quite frankly make your pregnancy experience miserable.

Even though finding a therapist who specializes in prenatal massage might be a difficult task, you should be cautious not to compromise the health of yourself and the unborn baby's well being by settling for an optional therapist.

In essence, do not assume that any and every massage therapists can accommodate you. Some might not have the experience and some might not feel comfortable accepting you as a patient at all.

Ask your potential masseuse or masseur if they have any experience dealing with pregnant clients. If they do not, they may probably be able to point you in the right direction.

Dealing with the third trimester

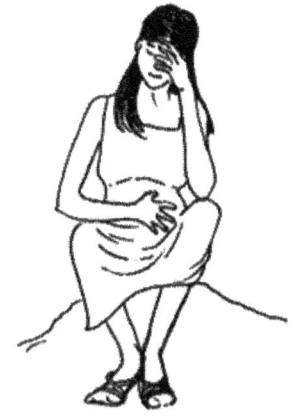

Just when you were beginning to enjoy the fun and excitement of the second trimester, you would suddenly discover that certain elements that you had felt in the first semester suddenly starts to creep in again.

There and then you ought to realize that you are actually already in the third trimester.

The third trimester of pregnancy can be a physically and emotionally challenging period for most would-be moms.

With your baby's size now at almost its largest, and constantly changing its position, your daily routine and sleep would be filled with gross discomfort and periodic misery.

Already rankled by intermittent sensations of your baby's movements in the third trimester, your body would soon be more pressured by additional experiences that would have brought about a more expanded series of changes to your physical structure.

These changes includes, but not limited to;

● *Continued breast growth*

By the middle of the third semester, your breast would have already have an additional 2 pounds (nearly 1 kilogram) of breast tissue added to the scale.

And as delivery approaches, your nipples could start leaking *colostrum* — the yellowish fluid that will nourish your baby during the first phases of his/her life.

● *Weight gain*

At minimum, your body would have also added an additional 25 to 35 pounds (about 11 to 16 kilograms) more than you did before pregnancy, as you approaches the end of your third trimester.

However, your baby would have accounted for some of the weight gain, in addition to the placenta, amniotic fluid, larger breasts, expanded uterus, extra fat stores, and increased blood and fluid volume.

● *Braxton Hicks contractions*

These contractions are usually the warm-ups and indication of the real thing thing to come. They're usually weak and come and go unpredictably.

However, the *Braxton Hicks Contractions* are usually more milder than True labor contractions, which are longer, stronger and closer together.

If you're having contractions that are painful or rapid, then it may be important for you to immediately contact your health care provider.

Because sometimes, the birth of your baby may be closer than you may have thought or may have been previously told.

● *Backaches*

As your baby continues to gain weight, pregnancy hormones would begin to relax the joints between the bones in your pelvic area. These changes can sometimes be burdensome on the structure of your back bone framing.

Therefore, you may need to take steps during your third trimester to alleviate these sort of discomforts.
For example, when you sit, choose chairs with good back support. Apply a heating pad or ice pack to the painful area.

Ask your partner for a massage. Wear low-heeled — but not flat — shoes with good arch support.

If the back pain doesn't go away or is accompanied by other signs and symptoms, contact your health care provider.

● *Shortness of breath*

As your uterus expands beneath your diaphragm, (the muscle just below your lungs), you might find that there may be some difficulty in breathing if you walk briskly or stand up for longer periods.

This usually occurs during the early stages of the third trimester, but may no longer be an issue when the baby settles deeper into your pelvis before delivery, around the end stages of the said trimester.

However, whenever you are hit with mild situations of short breathing, try to adopt a good posture and sleep with your upper body propped up on pillows to relieve pressure on your lungs.

● *Heartburn*

We had discussed the challenges of heartburn at length earlier in this book. But if you thought that the burning-stomach experiences of the first trimester had totally gone away, ... your are surely wrong.

Practically, during the third trimester, your growing uterus sometimes push your stomach out of its normal position, which is usually the main contributing factor to heartburn experience by pregnant women.

As in all cases, women in their third trimester (and even before) can keep stomach acid where it belongs by eating small meals and drink plenty of fluids between meals.

As always, you should avoid fried foods, carbonated drinks, citrus fruits or juices, and spicy foods.
If these tips don't help, ask your health care provider about antacids such as Rolaids and Andrews Liver Salts.

● *Swelling*
With a growing uterus now putting severe third-trimester pressure on the veins that returns blood from your feet and legs, you would notice that swollen feet and ankles may soon become an issue.

Additionally, swelling in your legs, arms or hands can place pressure on several nerves, causing tingling or numbness. As such, fluid retention and dilated blood vessels might leave your face and eyelids puffy, especially in the morning.

To reduce swelling, you may have to lie down frequently or use a footrest. You might even need to elevate your feet and legs while you sleep. It can also help to swim or simply stand in a pool.

● *Frequent urination*
You may not like this but as your baby moves deeper into your pelvis, you'll begin to feel more pressure on your

bladder. As such, you might find yourself urinating more often, even during the night.

This extra pressure might also cause you to leak urine — especially when you laugh, cough or sneeze.

But if you're worried about leaking urine in such cases, panty liners may very well save you some embarrassment.

Most importantly, you must continuously watch for signs of a *urinary tract infection*, which is self diagnose if you are urinating even more than usual, feeling a burning sensation during urination, cold sweating, an unexplained fever, abdominal pain and/or a piercing backache.

If left untreated, urinary track infections can increase the risk of pregnancy complications, and can even be passed on to your unborn baby during delivery.

● *Vaginal discharge*
Potentially heavy vaginal discharge is usually common at the later end of pregnancy. But if you saturate a panty liner within a few hours or wonder if the discharge is leaking amniotic fluid, you should contact your health care provider.

● *Spider veins, varicose veins and hemorrhoids*
As you progress further into your third trimester, increased blood circulation may cause tiny red veins, known as spider veins, to appear on your skin, in addition to a stream of blue and reddish lines beneath the surface of the skin *(varicose veins)*, particularly in the legs.

These *varicose veins* can also become a problem in your rectum, as hemorrhoids may more than likely begin to add itself to your list of pregnancy complications.

83

If you have painful varicose veins, elevate your legs and wear support stockings.

To prevent the bleeding effects of hemorrhoids, you may need to make some efforts to avoid constipation by including plenty of fiber in your diet and drink lots of fluids.

Constipation and Pregnancy: *How to Avoid it*

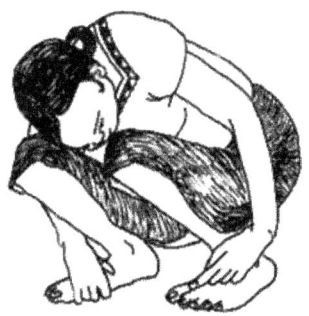

Nearly half of all the women who are pregnant, suffers from constipation during their pregnancy.

As with all symptoms of pregnancy, there is also a reason for constipation.

When you are pregnant your body creates a substance called *progesterone* which in turns relaxes the muscles of the bowels and causes your digestive tracks to work much slower. In essence, your digestive track works slower to make sure your body effectively absorbs the nutrients from your food for your baby.

However, while this process may benefit the baby, it can nonetheless create constipation problems for the pregnant mother, which if it not kept under control, can lead to hemorrhoids.

Nonetheless, there are some steps that you can take to help avoid constipation throughout your pregnancy.

First of all, make sure you included plenty of fiber in your diet. Fiber absorbs water and can help to soften your stools and speed their passage.
Additionally, you should eat plenty of high fiber foods like whole grain cereal and oatmeal.

Instead of eating white bread with your sandwiches, eat whole grain breads, and remember to add some oat bran to your cereals or yogurt.

Fresh fruits are also an excellent way to get your fiber in.

Melons and plums have a high amount of fiber in them as well as dried fruits like figs, raisins, apricots and of course the well known favorite, prunes.

For centuries, prunes and prune juice have been known to have a laxative effect and will help keep things moving properly in your body. Hence, you can aim to eat at least 25 to 30 grams of fiber a day.

You can tell you are getting enough fiber if your stools are large and soft and you aren't straining to pass them.
Keep in mind though that too much fiber can lead to diarrhea which can in turn lead to dehydration. Therefore, you should not over do the fiber in your diet.

Drinking plenty of fluid will also help you combat constipation.

Fluids help keep digestive products moving through your system. So it is very important for you to drink at least six to eight glasses of water a day, especially if you are increasing your intake of fiber.

This is because your body needs water to soak up the fiber; - otherwise it can cause more constipation.

You should also make sure you are eating an adequate dose of yogurt if you can.

Yogurt has a bacteria called *acidophilus* that helps stimulate the intestinal bacteria to break down food better.

Prenatal products can also lead to constipation.

Some of the prenatal content that women take usually contain a lot of iron which can play a big part in constipation.

Conclusively, you should simply avoid foods such as white bread, white rice, bananas and some cereals, especially corn flakes, since they can all lead to constipation.

But if all of the above fails, give your doctor a call to see if there is something you can take to help keep you regulated.

Most doctors will allow you to take *Metamucil* to help keep things moving.

Constipation is never pleasant but during pregnancy it can be even extra uncomfortable.

However, constipation may only one of the various and many health concerns that you may need to focus on during your third trimester.

Other health situations may include incidents of increased hypertension, in addition to gestational diabetes, which we may discuss hereafter.

Gestational Diabetes

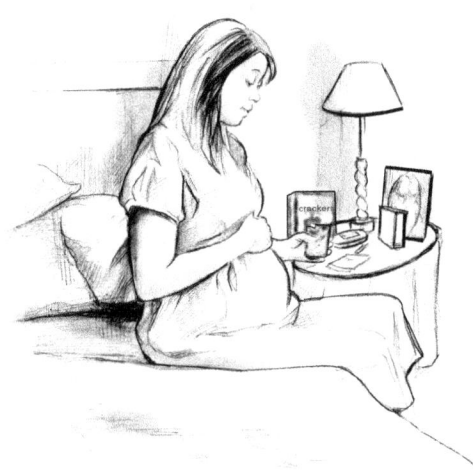

Gestational diabetes is one of the most common pregnancy complications that women face, and generally occurs when women who are not diabetic, suddenly develop very high blood sugar levels during their pregnancy.

It is not really known what can cause gestational diabetes. But it is widely believed that it is caused by pregnancy-related factors such as the presence of *Human Placenta Lactogen* (in pregnant women) which interferes with the susceptible insulin receptors, resulting in them not functioning properly. This in turn can cause inappropriately elevated blood sugar levels.

Some experts say that overweight women have a higher risk of developing gestational diabetes, but there is not much evidence to support this.

What is known about gestational diabetes is that one of the only cures is to deliver the baby. Because after delivery, your blood sugar level will go back down to normal.

The most common treatment for gestational diabetes during pregnancy has been insulin shots. This is usually apply daily to a pregnant woman, just as if she was suffering from diabetes.

Some women find though that by changing their diet, they are able to manage their gestational diabetes without having to give themselves a shot of insulin.

If you are looking to make dietary changes, your doctor will probably refer you to a nutritionist.

They will look at several factors when designing a meal plan for you.

First they will look at your weight before you got pregnant and how much you have gained since then. Next they will look at your activity level and your blood level. Then they will work with you to design an eating plan that has just the right amount of carbohydrates.

Some of the guidelines you should follow are to spread your carbs out throughout the day by eating three small meals and two to four snacks.

Breakfast might be a meal where you will want to eat less carbs since they can cause your blood sugar to rise quickly. Instead, you should eat a protein filled breakfast with eggs, or even meat.

Giving up sweets is one of the best things you can do if you have been diagnosed with gestational diabetes, as it will make your meal plan much easier to follow.

It is also important that you do not skip meals or try going on a low carb diet. This is going to cause your blood levels to fall to low levels and can leave you exhausted and legatheric.

Chances are that you will have to test your blood sugar levels regularly to make sure you are at a safe reading.

In other cases, some women are so sensitive that they can tell when their levels are low and would not necessarily depend upon a scientific instrument to alert them, before taking corrective measures.

Not taking the steps to keep your gestational diabetes under control would not only put you at a risk of developing type 2 diabetes's later in life, but you will also be putting the life of your baby at risk.

Babies born from moms who were diagnosed with gestational diabetes tend to be larger than those who aren't.

Most doctors will not let a woman go past her due date if she has gestational diabetes; - and a few will not even let them go as far as their due date before inducing them.

After all, larger babies could mean more delivery complications and would increase your chance of a c- section.

Choosing foods with a low GI (glycaemic index) will also help you to manage your gestational diabetes. That's because low-GI foods take longer for your body to digest. Glucose is released more slowly into your bloodstream.

Some examples of food with a low GI are: pasta made with durum wheat flour, apples, oranges, pears, peaches, beans and lentils, sweetcorn and porridge.

Gestational diabetes is so common today that no one would discern you if you say you have it.

But if you are eating a healthy diet and is watching your sugar level, then you will be able to control your blood sugar count and continue with a perfect pregnancy, and not having to be worried about gestational diabetes.

What Should I Do if The Baby Stops Moving?

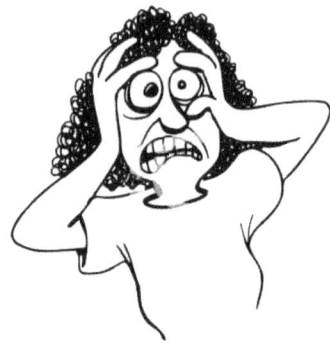

During the final stages of your third trimester, movement is an important sign that the fetus is doing well.

As your pregnancy progresses and your fetus gets larger and larger, the type of movement can change.

Instead of your fetus punching you or doing flips, the baby may roll more or stick an arm or leg out during the third trimester.

You should always pay attention to these movements. Even if your fetus is not moving as much as normal, keep track of its movements.

However, since there are many ways by which you can count fetal movement; you should ask your doctor or provider how he/she wants you to count.

But if you suspects that there is seemingly no movement, you can try a simply housewife trick to make a preliminary assessment of your baby's well being.

All you have to do is simply eat a meal and then lie down on your left side for a long while. If the fetus does not move around 10 times in the next two hours, you should promptly call or visit your health care provider.

If the fetus is not moving, your doctor will order a non-stress test, a contraction stress test, or a biophysical profile (BPP).

Third Trimester Health Readiness

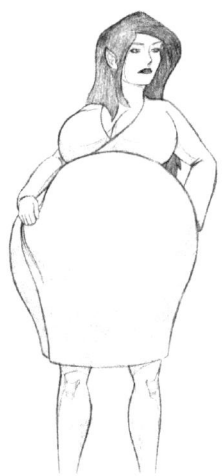

Even thought the latter part of the third trimester marks the finish of fetal development, and the concluding phase of your pregnancy, that does not mean that you should abandon the care and health practices necessary to secure the health of yourself and baby.

At this stage, you may want to void long car trips and airplane flights, if possible.

Your doctor will generally permit you to travel by air until 32 to 34 weeks of your pregnancy, unless you are at high risk for premature labor.
After that time, most airlines may not let you board the flight if you appear obviously pregnant because of the possibility of an unexpected delivery on the plane.

If you must travel though, stretch your legs and walk around at least every hour or two.

If you will be away from home for a long time, your doctor may recommend a local obstetrician where you are visiting for you to contact. Be sure to take a copy of your prenatal records with you.

If you must travel by car, lap and shoulder belts should be worn at all times when riding in a motor vehicle, particularly in the front seat. Being an unrestrained passenger during a major automobile accident is dangerous, whether or not you are pregnant.

If you are working, pregnancy *(even at the latter part of your third trimester)* is usually not affected by most occupations.
But if your job position becomes challenging for your pregnancy, you can ask an understanding employer to consider reassigning you to a position that involves less risk. However employers are not under any obligation to do so.

In other cases, you may need to consider proceeding on maternity leave early if you are working in an environment that is overwhelmed with occupational hazards such as an office that allows prolonged exposure to lead-based paints, working in a poorly ventilated setting with noxious fumes *(anesthetic gases, volatile chemicals)*, and unregulated radiation exposure.

Your own health and personal safety factors can also require that you cease any sort of work whatsoever.

This entails scenarios where certain obstetrical conditions may require compulsory bedrest during pregnancy, such as preterm labor, incompetent cervix, *placenta previa*, and *preeclampsia*.

But if you are not impeded by any of these conditions or is faced with any other health complications, then it should be ok for you to be in employment even up to your day of delivery.

Preparing for your expected baby

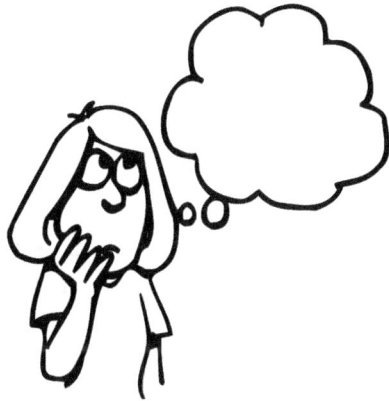

As your baby's due date draws near, you may be feeling a range of emotions.

It is normal to feel a mix of excitement, impatience and anxiety.

A really effective way to mentally prepare yourself for labour is to learn as much about the process as possible. As they say, knowledge is power.

The more you can understand about the child-birthing process, the more confident and empowered you will feel when the time actually arrives.

Nonetheless, you can better prepare yourself by considering the following; -

1 - Learn from other women experiences.
Ask a few friends or family members about their experiences.

While every woman's labour experiences are different, there may still be many similarities that you can learn from.

2. Make a birth plan

An essential way to prepare for your labour is to develop a birth plan. Your plan should include how you ideally want to deliver your little one *(vaginally or by Cesarean)* and where you want to deliver *(depending on your doctor and the hospital, your choices generally include a private hospital, public hospital or birthing centre)*.

It is also important to decide who you want by your side throughout the birth process. Your support person(s) should be a master of providing firm hand-holding and positive affirmations.

Bear in mind that your plan is really just a useful guide for how you would ideally like your birthing experience to be.

And, although your healthcare provider will try to stick to your goals as much as possible, there are certain situations where it may be necessary to deviate from the plan. As such, it is always best to have a flexible approach to your labour to avoid any disappointment. After all, the main aim is to have a safe and ideal delivery.

3. Decide on your preferred pain relief

It is difficult to predict just how painful labour will be for you as each person has a different pain threshold. However, child-birthing is generally a painful *(and often lengthy)* process.

While early labour pain has been described as 'severe menstrual-type cramping', the discomfort during the pushing stage has been delicately depicted as 'an excruciating stretching and burning sensation in the groin area'.

Even though the potential for pain during labour might concern you, bear in mind that pain is gain – and with each push and contraction, your little baby is one step closer to being born.

However, there are several pain management options that can be made available to you while you are in labour, and you should be able to choose to use a combination of these.

Some non-medication comfort measures include the use of hot and cold packs, lower back massage and walking.
Relaxation by way of meditation and breathing exercises are effective for some women.

Many women also find that water therapy by bath or shower is a useful method in helping to ease the discomfort of labour.

For many mums-to-be, pain may not be adequately controlled by natural measures alone.

If this occurs, there are several medications available to you, such as an *epidural*.

An *epidural* is a regional nerve block that involves injecting an anaesthetic into the lower back and the lining of the spinal cord. It provides effective pain relief by causing reduced sensation from the waist down; the amount of medication administered can be regulated according to your needs.

The main drawbacks of using an epidural are that it may make it more difficult to push the baby out and it can also cause a severe drop in blood pressure.

Narcotic analgesics (such as *pethidine* or *morphine*) are other medications which may be given during labour for pain relief. These medications act on your whole body to reduce pain and discomfort.

They don't usually slow labour down or interfere with contractions but they can cause drowsiness and nausea for the mother.

4. Stay active

Regular exercise is an ideal way to help strengthen your muscles and prepare your body for the stress of childbirth. Exercise can also increase your endurance, which will come in handy if you have a long labour.

However, before you begin any exercise during pregnancy, it's a good idea to talk to your doctor about what he/she considers as a safe regimen for you, given your pre-pregnancy fitness level and your health status.

You can also start to physically prepare 'down there' by doing pelvic exercises.

Pelvic floor exercises help to strengthen the structures supporting the uterus and bladder, and studies have shown that women who perform them regularly during the last few months of pregnancy are more likely to reduce the length of their second stage of labour *(the pushing stage)*, thereby minimizing labour discomfort.

As if this isn't incentive enough, regular pelvic floor exercises also help reduce the development of urinary incontinence after birth.

5. Organise the house

Although it may be hard to imagine, it won't be long before you have to bring your beloved one home with you, or taking a temporary stay-over regimen with them by your mom's house.
But while you are waiting for this to happen, there are several ways you can prepare yourself on the domestic front.

Therefore, to prevent the need for unnecessary shopping expeditions when your baby first comes home, stock up on newborn nappies and other basic essentials.

Wash the cot sheets now so they are ready to go when you need them.

If you feel up to it, cook and freeze a few meals in advance for you and your partner (you will really appreciate this once baby is here).

If you won't feel up to cooking yourself, ask a family member (who is probably willing to help in any way) to come over and help you prepare the meals and do some washing daily.

6. Pack your bag
As you get closer to the 36-week mark, it's time to start packing your hospital bag.

After all, it would be a disaster to be scrambling around for lollies and slippers in between contractions.

In choosing what to wear during labour, it is best to remember three main principles: comfort is crucial; access is vital, so your midwife or doctor can check your progress regularly; and labour can be messy; - so only bring items that you don't mind ruining.

Some women choose to wear an oversized nightshirt during their labour, while others opt to wear a hospital gown or nothing at all!

Other essential items for your hospital stay include toiletries, a couple of nighties with easy front access for breastfeeding, maternity pads (catered for heavy bleeding) and comfy lounge clothes for during the days.

Large granny panties, nursing bras, vaginal health wash tubes, health soap, and other self care products may also be necessary to pack.

You will also need diapers, wipes, and some clothing for your baby to wear after delivery and when you have to leave the hospital.

Don't feel pressured to have every baby product you'll ever need. You can wait on some items.

Stressing out yourself to get a perfect hospital list may not be good for a healthy delivery.

Furthermore, you are not moving into the hospital to take up residence. So why would you need to pack a large suitcase anyway?

Days away from delivery

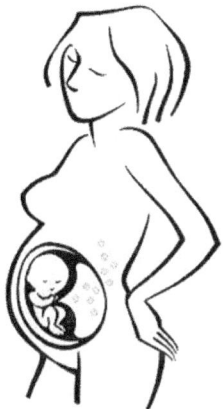

No one can predict with certainty when labour will actually begin. The due date that your doctor gives to you is usually just a point of reference.

As such, it is normal for labor to start as early as three weeks before that date or as late as two weeks after it.

Actually, your body would have started preparations for labor up to a month before you give birth, and you may not had a clue of what's going on — or you may begin to notice new symptoms as your due date draws near.

● *Your baby "drops."*
If this is your first pregnancy, you may feel what's known as "lightening" a few weeks before labor starts. You might sense a heaviness in your pelvis as this happens and would notice less pressure just below your ribcage, making it easier to catch your breath.

● *Braxton Hicks contractions intensifies*
More frequent and intense *Braxton Hicks contractions* can signal pre-labor, during which your cervix ripens and the

stage is set for true labor. Some women experience a crampy, menstrual-like feeling during this time.

Sometimes, as true labor draws near, the Braxton Hicks contractions become relatively painful and strike as often as every ten to 20 minutes, making you wonder whether true labor has started.

But if the contractions don't get longer, stronger, and closer together and cause your cervix to dilate progressively, then what you're feeling is probably a so-called false labor.

● *Your cervix starts to change.*
In the days and weeks before delivery, changes in the connective tissue of your cervix will cause it to soften.

Braxton Hicks contractions may have already done some of the preliminary work of thinning and perhaps opening your cervix a bit. *(If you've given birth before, your cervix is more likely to dilate a centimeter or two before labor starts, but keep in mind that even being 40 weeks pregnant with your first baby and 1 centimeter dilated is no guarantee that labor is imminent.)*

When you're at or near your due date, your practitioner may do a vaginal exam during your prenatal visit to see whether your cervix has started to change.

● *You pass your mucus plug or notice "bloody show."*
You may pass your mucus plug *(the small amount of thickened mucus that has sealed your cervical canal during the last nine months)* if your cervix begins to efface significantly or dilate as you get close to labor.

The plug may come out in a lump or as increased vaginal discharge over the course of several days.

The mucus may be tinged with brown, pink, or red blood, which is why it's referred to as "bloody show."
Having sex or a vaginal exam can also disturb your mucus plug and cause you to see some blood-tinged discharge, even when labor actually isn't going to start in the next few days.

● *Your water breaks.*
Most women start having regular contractions before their water breaks, but in some cases, the water breaks first.

In actuality, when the fluid-filled amniotic sac surrounding your baby ruptures, fluid leaks from your vagina. And whether it comes out in a large gush or a small trickle, it is surely time to call your doctor or midwife, or immediately start your trip to the hospital. Because when this happens, labour usually follows soon after.

Arriving at the hospital

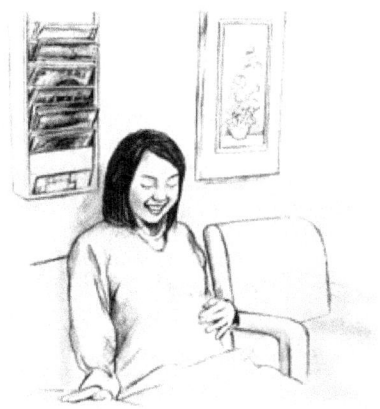

Even in cases where the water bag had not been ruptured as yet, most women would simply proceed to the hospital once they are experiencing excruciating labour pains or if they are of the view that they are ready for delivery.

However, turning up at the hospital does not mean that they would immediately admit you or roll you into a delivery room. The hospital would first need to evaluate your health condition upon arrival so as to determine whether you are indeed in labour.

As such, when you first arrive at the hospital reception: - a nurse will examine you, take your blood pressure and possibly a urine sample, and consult with your physician to determine whether you will be admitted.

You may need to stay in the reception area for some time while the doctor(s) determine the intensity of your labor. This can sometimes seem like a tedious and tormenting process especially if the cramps and labour pains have worsened, while you wait.

Nonetheless, you may still have to exercise some patience while your doctor makes his/her evaluation.

To check your baby's heart rate, a fetal monitor will be applied. The nurse will give you an expandable belt for use with the fetal monitor that you will need to put around your stomach under your hospital gown.

If you are not admitted on your first visit, do not be disappointed ; - it is very common for women to experience symptoms of labor but not being ready to deliver.

In such a case, you may had probably experienced a false start and would have been advised to return home or to be kept for further assessment.

But if you are indeed in labour and your health care provider determined that you may be actually ready for delivery, then some forms may be completed to admit you into the hospital. Upon admission, you can then proceed to discuss your birth plan with your nurse and doctor

Preparing for delivery

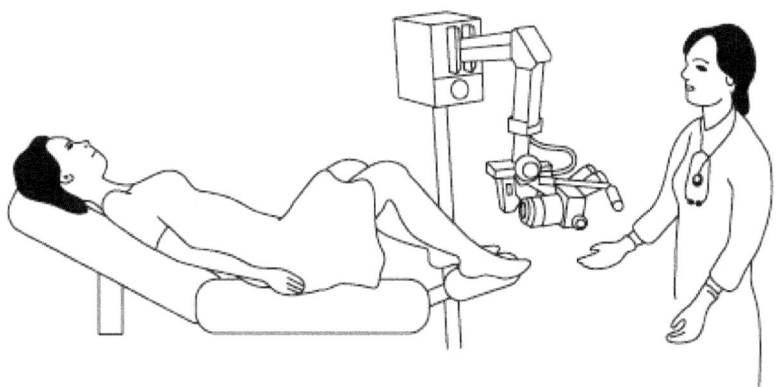

In order for you to be admitted and be prepared for delivery of your baby, you would have had already past the stage of early labour *(which usually occurs prior to arriving at the hospital)*.

During early labor, your cervix will begin to dilate. You'll feel mild contractions during early labor.
They will typically last 30 to 90 seconds and come at regular intervals. Near the end of early labor, your contractions will likely be less than five minutes apart.

As your cervix begins to open, you might notice a brown or blood-tinged discharge from your vagina, as we had discussed earlier in this book.

This discharge is likely the mucus plug that blocks the cervical opening, also known as *bloody show*.

Early labor is unpredictable. For first-time moms, the average length of early labor is 6 to 12 hours. It can however become much shorter for subsequent deliveries.

However, you would have already gone past your early labour stage in order for the doctor to admit you for delivery.

And once you are in the delivery room, it would mean that you are in *Active Labour;* - which is time for the real work to begin.

During active labor, your cervix will dilate to 10 centimeters (cm). Your contractions will become stronger, longer, closer together and regular. Your legs might cramp, and you might feel nauseous.

You might feel your water break — if it hasn't already, in addition to an increasing pressure in your back as well.

Active labor often lasts up to eight hours. For some women, active labour can lasts for longer hours, while for others (especially those who've had a previous vaginal delivery) it can be much shorter.

In the meantime, try a breathing and relaxation technique to combat your growing discomfort. Use what you have learned in this book, or from your maternal classes, or ask your health care team for suggestions.
Nonetheless, to promote comfort during active labour, you can:

- Change positions
- Take a warm shower or bath
- Take a walk, and stopping to breathe through contractions
- Have a gentle massage between contractions.

After a while you would begin to go into an advance stage (first stage) of active labour known as *Transition*, and which would give you a sudden urge to push as your cervix becomes ready to commence delivery of your baby.

If you feel the urge to push but you're not fully dilated, your health care provider might ask you to hold back.

In essence, pushing too soon could cause your cervix to swell, which might delay delivery.

As such, you should simply pant or blow your way through the contractions.

Delivering your baby

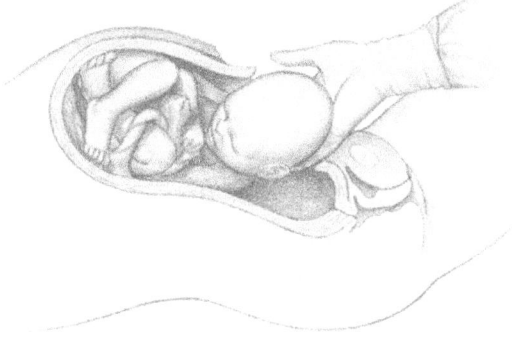

You'll deliver your baby during the second stage of labor, which can be a few minutes from the first stage or transition stage.

It can take from a few minutes up to a few hours or more to push your baby into the world, or even longer for first-time moms and women who've had an epidural.

But once the delivery process has started, the best thing for you to do is; - Push!

You might be encouraged to push with each contraction to speed the process, or you might take it more slowly, letting nature do the work until you feel the urge to push.

When you push, don't hold tension in your face. Bear down and concentrate on pushing where it counts.

Experiment with different positions until you find one that feels best. As a matter of fact, you can push while squatting, sitting, kneeling — even on your hands and knees.

Between contractions, you'll need to conserve your energy and rest up for the next round since pushing is labour (and delivery) intensive.

If you become exhausted, your practitioner may suggest you stop pushing for a couple of contractions to regain some strength.

At first, it may seem like you're pushing for nothing, but soon you'll be rewarded with results. You'll need to keep in mind, though, that pushing is a two steps forward, one step backward process — so don't become frustrated when your baby's head crowns (shows) and then disappears again.

At some point, you might be asked to push more gently, not to push anymore, or simply to slow down.

Slowing down gives your vaginal tissues time to stretch rather than tear.

But with a few more additional pushing efforts, your delivery ordeal would soon yield its desired result, as your baby's head would be the first part of his/ her tiny structure to make its way out.

Once your baby's head has eased its way out, your practitioner will suction out any mucus from the nose and mouth, then help guide the shoulders and torso out and those cute little legs.

You'll probably be able to hold your baby right away and you'll revel in that first lusty cry.

Shortly after delivery, your baby's umbilical cord will be cut by your practitioner, and the delivery process will then take it final phase.

It's also likely that your newborn will get a brisk rubdown, be wrapped (and get a cute little hat) to prevent heat loss, and have ointment placed in his or her eyes to prevent infection.

For health reasons, and to help him/her to better adjust to breathing and dwelling in the open world, your baby would be washed or wiped and place in an incubator for as little as a few hours to as much as a few days *(or even for a few weeks if survival challenges are discovered)*

You may not be able to take possession of your baby until your health care provider feels that it is safe to remove the child from incubation or feels it is safe enough to dwell in normal environmental conditions.

● Delivery of the Placenta

While your newborn baby would have been out enjoying a good bath (cleansing) or being placed in the incubator, the delivery process for you is not yet completely over.

Your healthcare team would have been busy with the final phase of the childbirth process, which is; - removing the *Placenta*.

The placenta, also known as afterbirth, is a combination of soft tissues which had been providing bed and board for your baby for most of his or her stay in your uterus. Its delivery is necessary in order to bring an end of the birth process.

This last stage of childbirth usually lasts anywhere from between five to 20 minutes or more, in the delivery room.
Mild contractions that last about a minute each and which you may not even notice will help separate the placenta from the uterine wall and move it through the birth canal so that you can push it out.

Your practitioner may help speed up the process by putting gentle pressures on your uterus.

Once the placenta is delivered your practitioner will clean and stitch up any vaginal tears that you may have.

After delivery of the placenta (or the after birth) you'll notice some bloody vaginal discharge (called lochia) that may be comparable to a heavy period, while you may start experiencing chills.

You may also most likely be feeling hungry and thirsty *(especially if labour was long and you weren't able to eat or drink)* while having a wide range of emotions — especially relief, elation, and impatience to get your hands on the baby.

But as it is, the entire birth process would have now been over, and you would have been escorted to a room to get yourself cleaned up and then assign a bed to rest, prior to reuniting with your baby.

Conclusion: *connecting with your newborn*

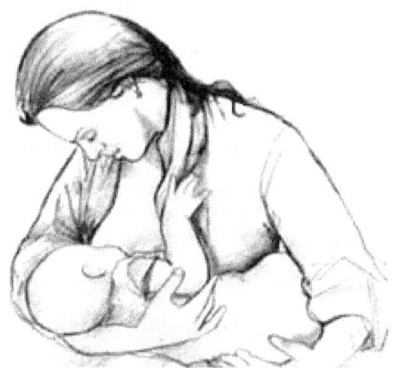

After reuniting with your newborn, you would suddenly find yourself juggling between congratulatory phone calls, bedside visits, and a struggle for privacy with your baby, even before you leave the hospital.

But regardless of all the excitement and visits in the air, bonding with your baby is an important process that you won't want to be derailed.

Bonding simply refers to the intense attachment you develop with your baby.

It's the feeling that makes you want to shower him/ her with love and affection, or throw yourself in front of a speeding truck to protect him/ her.

For some parents, this takes place within the first few days – or even minutes – of birth. For others, it may take a little longer.

But regardless of how long it would take, your newborn is now a special gift of life that is as a result of your enduring pregnancy.

Hence, it will be time to say goodbye to nine months of agony, and welcome to a lifetime of joy.

Congratulations on a well-managed maternity period and a successful delivery!!

The end

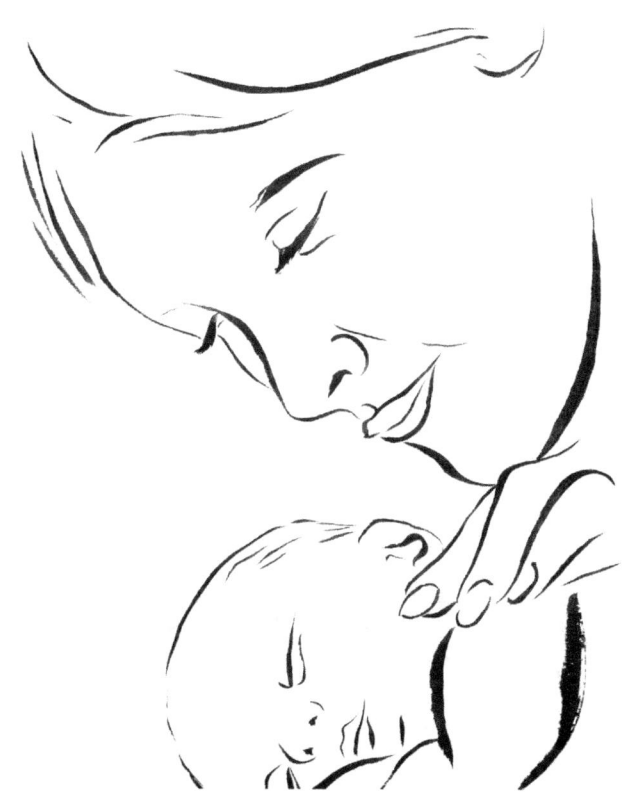

Recommended reading and other quality sources of information for pregnant mothers

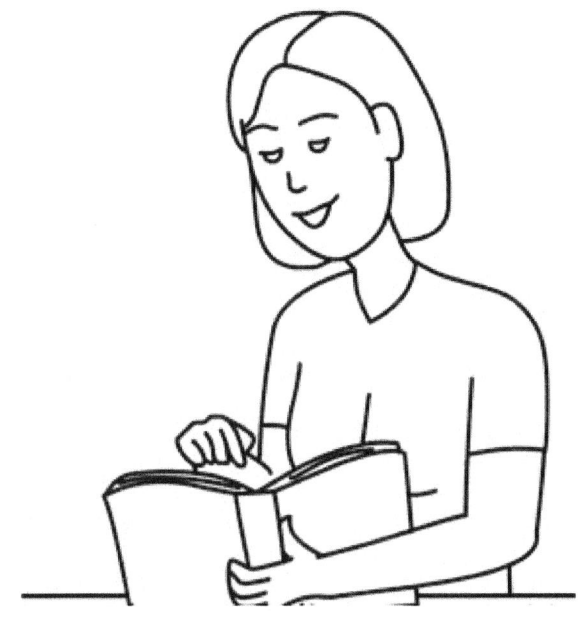

http://www.mayoclinic.com/

http://www.babycenter.com/

http://www.babycenter.co.uk/

http://www.whattoexpect.com/

www.webmd.com

www.parents.com

http://www.healthline.com/